Faith, Hope, and Healing

Faith, Hope, and Healing

Inspiring Lessons Learned from
People Living with Cancer

Bernie Siegel, M.D.
and
Jennifer Sander

WILEY

John Wiley & Sons, Inc.

Published by John Wiley & Sons, Inc., Hoboken, New Jersey
Published simultaneously in Canada

Library of Congress Cataloging-in-Publication Data:
Siegel, Bernie S.
    Faith, hope, and healing : inspiring lessons learned from people living with cancer / Bernie Siegel and Jennifer Sander.
        p.   cm.
    Includes index.
    ISBN 978-0-470-28901-3 (cloth)
        1. Cancer—Psychological aspects.   2. Medicine, Psychosomatic.   I. Sander, Jennifer Basye, 1958–   II. Title.
    [DNLM: 1. Neoplasms—psychology—Personal Narratives. 2. Faith Healing—Personal Narratives. 3. Survivors—psychology—Personal Narratives. QZ 200 S571f 2009]
    RC262.S477   2009
    616.99'4—dc22
                                                                                    2008055871

Printed in the United States of America
10 9 8 7 6 5 4 3 2 1

To my creators: those of a higher order whom we can only sense as being present; and to my parents, my wife Bobbie, our five children and eight grandchildren, and innumerable divine creatures of varying species who have shared their lives with us.

Contents

Part Two: HOPE

Part Three: HEALING

Acknowledgments

I'd like to thank Andrea Hurst and Jennifer Sander for their devotion to the book and for guiding me through the process of creating it, and to Tom Miller at John Wiley and Sons for his support of my work and editorial direction with this book. Special thanks to Samantha Layne and Amberly Finarelli for their assistance.

Introduction

After countless years of helping people participate in the process of healing their lives and curing their bodies when they have been diagnosed with cancer, I can tell you that I have seen the power of faith, hope, and healing, and what they can accomplish. These three states of grace have taught me that all the side effects of cancer are not by definition bad. So-called curses can become blessings, and an illness can help us come alive as human beings. Many people see their disease as a wake-up call that inspired them to literally begin their life anew. The side effects of cancer can become the labor pains by which we give birth to ourselves and the lives we were meant to live. The side effects empower us to nourish our lives, just as hunger forces us to seek nourishment for our bodies.

In the following pages, I will share with you the inspiring stories of those who have experienced cancer, and in their own way found deeper faith, hope, and healing—and even joy through the process. If you or someone you love has been diagnosed with cancer, these stories will encourage and help you to develop attitudes and behaviors that survivors share, while also offering you a myriad of ways to get through this difficult time and discover the gifts that cancer can bring into your life. After each entry, I will share my reflections about the lessons that can be learned and the wisdom derived from experiencing these stories.

Why collect these stories? Why do I feel it is truly educational and healing to read the stories of others who have gone through similar ordeals? To put it simply, it is because the tourists cannot help the natives. What I mean is, those who have experienced a diagnosis of cancer can help you to cope with and triumph over yours. What can you learn from people like Carol Westfahl, Tom Martin, Jane Goldman, and the many other brave individuals whose stories are included here? You can learn the enormous healing power of art, the amazing transformation that journaling can produce, and the spiritual resources available to us all. Each person shares how their desire, intention, determination, and willingness to survive led them to become an active participant in their life and health. In all cases, the decision to participate and take responsibility was a true turning point in their life.

Faith is needed to survive. Life is full of obstacles that make it difficult and sometimes seem meaningless, but faith will help you to find support and meaning. As you adjust to the changes of your day-to-day life after your diagnosis, or the diagnosis of a loved one, you will find that faith is a strong component in helping to pull you through. There is a reason God didn't make a perfect world—perfection would make our lives meaningless. We would never have the opportunity to grow and appreciate life's little gifts and miracles if everything were already perfect.

Faith and spirituality relate to the wonder and creation of life. But what you have faith in is the key. Just as you have a remote control to select channels, you use your mind to select what messages you are open to and where your faith is placed. When you have faith, your actions become creative. You can trust in what comes your way and use it to better your life and the lives of those around you.

"Hope," Emily Dickinson wrote, "is the thing with feathers, that perches in the soul, and sings the tune without the words, and never stops at all." How can anyone live without hope? One oncologist, giving a protocol with four chemotherapeutic agents which began with the letters EPO and H, realized that if he turned the letters around they spelled HOPE. So he began to call his therapy program the HOPE Protocol. While others gave the EPOH Protocol, he found that he had more patients responding positively to his therapy even though they were all given the same drugs and dosage.

When we feel no hope, because of the words of doctors or others, we are more likely to die because of what this does to our attitude, immune function, and various hormone levels. Hope is real and not necessarily related to statistics. Words can help heal us by focusing our beliefs and mind on messages of love and encouragement. With renewed hope, joy can appear.

Joy is found in the relationships with those we love, whether it is with our family, friends, or beloved pets. Our relationships help keep us alive and make our lives meaningful. Often people try to find happiness through material things or by being a financial success, and then find that success does not make them happy. I say joy and success are found when you do what makes you happy.

A cancer diagnosis gives many people permission to live life to the fullest. The pain of cancer helps redefine them by granting them the permission to do the things they were either too busy or simply afraid to do. The disease frees them to reclaim their true identity and reminds them of the freedom of choice that is theirs and always has been. I hope those of you who read their stories will learn from them and not wait for, or need, a disease to enlighten you.

Remember, what we are talking about is healing your life and focusing your life's energy on healing. Healing and curing are two very separate processes. I know it to be true that when you heal your life, you may experience a cure as a side effect. But when you focus only on the mechanical aspects of treatment and curing your disease while neglecting yourself and your life, you are expending your energy by engaging in a struggle, and your life becomes more like a war than a process of healing.

Medical treatment can be seen not just as an attempt to not die, but as a part of the healing process, too. When you heal your life, you free yourself of the old wounds accumulated over a lifetime.

In a sense, you reparent yourself and bring forth the divine child within you. When the change occurs, your entire body feels the love you now have for life, and it strives to keep you alive and eliminate any afflictions that threaten your life.

Remember, your body loves you and knows how to heal, but it needs to know you love it and that you also love your life and the opportunities it provides you with. You are born with a potential to not just survive but to thrive. You deserve the opportunity to do this by healing the old wounds and moving on to a new life and journey with faith, hope, and joy as your companions.

I urge you to redirect your life toward enjoying the day instead of just doing your job, or fulfilling a role that someone else has assigned to you. As part of the healing process I have seen, people move, change jobs, get divorced, toss out their ties and jackets, or buy a house on the ocean. When people choose to live joyfully, as they were meant to do, it turns out they live longer, healthier, and happier lives. Let your inner light burn brightly and be a beacon for others. To do that, you must let your life shine. Some time ago a friend moved to Colorado after his cancer diagnosis because he was told he had a short time left to live and he'd always dreamed of living in the mountains. It was expected that he would die very soon. After some time, I hadn't heard anything from his family and began to wonder if they had forgotten to invite me to the funeral. I was upset and called them, only to have him answer the phone and say, "It was so beautiful here I forgot to die."

This book can offer you a gift, the encouragement and inspiration to eliminate fear from your life. When you heal your life and in the process bring faith, hope, and joy into your life, fear cannot exist. I know this to be true because I have lived and worked with many of these courageous people whose experiences you are about to witness. Their stories will teach you, as they have taught me, about our common strengths and how to live an authentic, joy-filled life.

PART ONE

Faith

God Handed Me a Gift

Angela Passidomo Trafford

How many times do I have to have cancer?! I stood in the center of my living room with the phone receiver still dangling in my hand and raged against God at the total unfairness and tragedy of my life. I'd just received two phone calls within minutes of each other. The first coldly informed me that, after years of international courtroom battles with my first husband, I'd lost custody of my three beloved boys. The second call, almost as cold, was from my doctor informing me that my breast cancer had returned.

What were my options? I had no money to continue fighting for custody. I didn't even have the money to go and see them. I saw no reason for a future, and I was in so much pain that I could no longer stand to be inside my own body. Suicide was an option. I realized in a moment of truth, though, that threatening suicide was yet another attempt to manipulate God to my own ends. My ego admitted defeat, and I got down on my knees in my living room and admitted that I wanted to live. I also admitted that I did not know how to live, that all my attempts at living life had ended in tragedy, pain, and illness. I let go of my life and asked God to show me how to live.

Without knowing exactly where I was going or why, I got into my car and began to drive aimlessly in a haze of fear and suffering. Fully alive to the realities of my life for perhaps the first time, I spotted a fortune-teller's sign and turned into the driveway. When this woman answered the door, she took one look at my face and said, "I don't know what has happened to you, but this will all turn around for you in the next few years." I hung on to her words as I headed back to the car and continued my aimless journey.

I ended up at the public library in my town, a spot I'd never before visited. As I wandered along the shelves, my eyes too glazed to pick out the titles of the books in front of me, the librarian approached me. In her hands she held a book—*Love, Medicine, and Miracles* by Bernie Siegel, M.D. She said, "Have you read this book?" I shook my head, no, I hadn't, and took the book she handed to me. However had she known that was what I needed at that moment? It was an amazing beginning to a journey of healing.

I wept as I read the book at home. Here were the answers I'd been seeking, and I knew this was the response to my prayers. God had handed me a great gift, he had answered me. The humility and gratitude were a welcome relief, a balm to my soul. It was a joy to look to God for help now instead of having to bluff my way through life, pretending to know it all. In the next few weeks, with the help of God, I began to take charge of my life and my health. My scheduled biopsy was three weeks away, and I planned to make real changes to myself before then.

I began rising at dawn and watching the first pink rays of sunlight sweeping the sky. I reached inside and thanked God for each new day, releasing tears of gratitude, which were followed by an immense rush of energy that was none other than the healing energy of hope. I'd take bike rides, fully alive to the moment like a child. After riding I would sit on my couch and practice the meditation and visualization exercises that Bernie had recommended in his book.

To my amazement one day, a visualization came forth from within myself of little birds eating golden crumbs; the little birds were the immune system cells and the crumbs were the cancer cells. I visualized the cancer in the form of golden crumbs, buttery and rich. I would follow this visualization by imagining a white light coming down through the top of my head, flowing throughout my entire body and healing me.

One morning after almost three weeks of biking and meditating, I sat down on the couch to begin my routine. As I began my visualization of the little white birds, something different happened. All of a sudden I felt the white light flow through the top of my head with tremendous force and energy. I can remember the exact experience—it was the experience of my duality as a human being. My heart pounded wildly as this tremendous heat and energy entered me. My rational mind was saying, "Get up! You are having a heart attack!" I ignored it calmly, not thinking of anything but simply letting myself go to the experience. I chose to let go and allow my being to become one with that beautiful light, that powerful energy.

Moments later I lay slumped on the couch. What a feeling—for the first time in my life my mind was free of all thought. For the first time in my life I experienced a deep, silent peace. It was like a smile in my heart. I knew, I just knew, that something wonderful had happened.

When my husband returned home that day, I told him what had happened and then shared with him my secret belief—that if another mammogram was taken, it would be clear. "They won't find anything there," I told him confidently.

I kept my doctor's appointment later that week. Before we began, my doctor came in with the previous mammogram in his hand, placing it on the light board so that I could see the cancerous dark shadow that lurked within. I said nothing about my healing experience to him, but I expressed no fear at the sight of the film. I was in a state of balance with myself, and I knew how it would turn out. The doctor left, I undressed, and the technician took a mammogram. I dressed again and waited for the doctor to come back and discuss the new pictures. But it was the technician who returned: "The doctor wants just one more mammogram."

Actually, the doctor wanted eight mammograms that day, before finally acknowledging what I already knew deep inside—that the cancer was gone. He was happy and excited for me, but mystified.

I told him about the little birds and the golden crumbs. I told him about the powerful white light. He looked into my eyes, took both my hands in his, and said with true sincerity, "Call it little birds, or call it what you will, but you are a very lucky woman."

BERNIE'S REFLECTION

Everything in the universe is subject to change, and everything is on schedule.

I would say Angela is not a lucky woman, she is an exceptional woman. Why call it luck? Why not give her the credit and learn from what she did and share her story with other patients? Between a painful custody battle and a life-threatening illness recurring, she saw very little in her life worth living for. It is only natural to feel this way. It was truly a miracle that Angela was able to find inspiration at the lowest point in her life. Rather than choose to lose her physical life, she chose to eliminate the life that was killing her, and in so doing she literally saved her own life. I always encourage people to never give up or forget the blessings that life still has to offer. To spend time thinking about what you are grateful for each day can help you survive. Your body needs to receive a "live" message so it, too, will fight for your life. We are capable of making genetic changes, as are bacteria, viruses, and plants when they are affected by antibiotics, vaccines, and droughts, and are still able to survive. Of course, it is easier for them to choose life because they do not have all the stress and problems people have.

Angela was more than lucky to achieve her outcome and survival. She did something powerful that made a difference in her healing. She accepted herself, her divine origin, and the power of inner peace to heal her life. She chose life rather than death despite cancer and divorce. As a result, her disease was cured as well. The doctor would have learned something powerful if he had asked Angela to tell her story so he could pass it on to other patients as a source of encouragement and hope.

After reading *Love, Medicine, and Miracles*, Angela began the journey of healing her body by healing her mind. The book may have inspired her, but she did the work that made the difference. We can coach others, but they need to show up for practice and rehearsals, or the best coaching in the world is ineffective. With her strong, positive attitude and faith in God, she found an exercise that helped to change her life. Angela's image of the birds feeding on the cancer gave her the reassurance she needed to know that everything was going to be all right. This peaceful image was not about killing the enemy and fighting a war, but about nourishment and healing.

I suggest you find a visual image that feels comfortable for you and provides you with hope and empowerment. I know a woman who had no results when she saw her white cells as vicious dogs eating her tumor, but when the tumor became a block of ice in her visualization, God's light melted it away.

Remember to live each day to the fullest, and like Angela did, take pleasure in simple activities that most people take for granted. When you listen to your inner self, all will be made clear to you.

A Snowy Quest

Barbara Hollace

Through the snow my husband and I drove to secure a piece of his life that would bring him comfort and joy. The winter had been harsh, weather and cancer coconspiring to present a spectacular grand finale.

Snow was piled up along the road as we began the long journey. The end was near and it was time to prepare for the farewell service. Our days were focused on my husband, Dalton, and granting his final wishes. A radio station "out in the boondocks" had agreed to make a copy of a special song for the funeral. It was important to him, and for me, because it was about granting his last request and giving him some control of his fading life.

This trip would parallel the path we had traveled thus far in our lives together. The cancer had drawn every ounce of energy from his body, and his system was barely functioning. A small spark of life remained. I knew it wasn't time to let go yet.

As we left the city, my gloved hands tightly gripped the steering wheel. Winter driving was beyond my comfort zone; in fact, it scared me to death. My life in recent years had been defined more by my fears than by reality, and so my forte had become slaying monsters at every turn. Our days were spent in deathly silence with few spoken words. There wasn't much more that could be said; we had made our peace. His sister would soon be arriving for her final visit. The inevitable was at hand. Clarity comes near the end of life's journey if we have the courage to open our eyes and really see the truth. This was as true for Dalton as it was for me.

Periodically I glanced at him in the passenger seat. He was shrinking away. The driver's seat was his place, not mine. Dalton was a professional truck driver who controlled large semis as if they were kiddy cars. Now he was no longer in the seat of control; his cancer had driven him from this position of power.

A vulnerability of my own spirit had taken over in the past weeks. I was so exhausted that I could hardly breathe. Tears flowed during the night hours, while my fears accompanied me by day as I worked to keep a paycheck coming in the door. Soon that would end, too. I could no longer juggle two jobs plus take care of him. My gas tank was empty. The hospice workers helped me shoulder the load, but I was his wife, who, for some reason, aspired to be Superwoman beneath my weary exterior.

There were moments of bitterness. I would continue to live and he would die. It made him angry. Dalton was only fifty-one and he was getting shortchanged. The passion of our love had been reduced to smoldering embers as we prepared for life's greatest test, staring death in the face. My emotions vacillated between victory and defeat. I was a recent law school graduate who loved studying and stretching my mind, but at times I felt guilty that it gave me so much pleasure. How could I be happy when he was sad? Joy and sorrow sat side by side in our car that day.

Silently we took a panoramic survey of our lives together. We each had experienced life intensely before our first encounter. Our memories could fill a scrapbook, and they would be the legacy he left behind.

Dalton had traveled the path of death before with his mother. Today he was the one in the passenger seat, and the view was different from there. He was no longer the driver, I was. Our lives and our safety were in my hands. It was a strange position of power for me. Too often I had willingly given the reins of control to someone else.

The past couldn't be changed, but each day was a small gift to celebrate. The time had arrived for me to take control not just of my life and future, but of this final journey together as well.

Few words were exchanged as the heat blasted inside the car and the cold tried to penetrate our cocoon. I drove cautiously as we left the civilized world behind and entered unknown territory. It was a living illustration of our lives. We were heading into uncharted waters or, in this case, snowbanks. Neither of us knew the way, only our final destination. We had traveled beyond our comfort zone and exchanged roles.

He had to trust me, and beyond that, I needed to trust myself and proceed with confidence. The landmarks looked familiar according to the directions we had been given. Ahead I saw a building that must be the radio station.

The music exchange was made quickly, a sudden ending for such a long trek. "No charge," was all they said. What was there to say, though, when you knew the purpose of the song? The tape that held such great significance was safely in my hand.

My life had become a treasure hunt. Sometimes I was given a clue to the next piece, but mostly I felt my way along in the dark. God alone knew the path that would bring this wild ride to an end. I chose to believe that God would remain with me, just as surely as my husband would soon leave me alone.

The cancer had taken its toll on me. Physically, I was run down. Emotionally, I was drained. Spiritually, only prayer held me together.

As we headed back to Spokane, my inner child wanted to run away and never return to our house of pain. My destiny was to face death's final hand and I could not figure out a way to avoid the confrontation.

My burden was twofold: watching him pull away from life, and keeping a secret in my heart. I'd learned that this stress had left an imprint on my body and soul. A doctor's appointment had revealed a small lump in my breast that would need to be monitored. There was no mistake about its location—the lump lived in my left breast over my heart, a testimony to all the unknowns in my life. Was it cancer? Had I been chosen to walk the same path to death's door?

I wouldn't add this burden to Dalton's weakened state. He needed to believe that I would be okay. I was a strong, courageous woman who had chosen to marry at the age of thirty, a woman who would be a widow three short years later. The author of my story had a twisted sense of humor.

As we drove home, our conversation ended. He was tired and soon fell asleep. Left alone with my own thoughts and feelings, I held back my tears. Again. I was getting good at this. "Breathe in hope, breathe out love" had been my mantra since his first surgery. Hope, love, and faith were the Three Musketeers who protected and guided me.

Throughout this journey when my heart asked, "Why?" my mind answered, "Why not? This is your path, your destiny. You have been given a gift that few are offered." With grace, and with time, I would be able to push past denial and anger, and accept God's gift.

God and I had our share of private conversations. On this day, God's message was resounding: "My child, I give you a glimpse of life's simplicity. Push pettiness aside. Life is short. Enjoy the moments you are given. Share your healing to bring hope to others. Your reward will be abundance in every way. There will be someone waiting for you on the other side of your grief. At the end of your loss, you will experience joy again."

I did not respond outwardly; the words echoed throughout my mind instead. We were near the city and close to home. Our home was an apartment that had become both a refuge and a prison. Death was the jailer who held the keys to our exit from this place.

Dalton's body would be free of cancer and mine would awaken to a new dawn. My tumor was benign. The responsibility of his life would no longer be mine. In time the emptiness would be filled with joyful purpose, and someday even laughter would return to my lips.

I felt God holding our hands as Dalton slipped beyond my reach. My husband's final hours were quiet as he finally found his peace. At the end, it had been just the two of us. The memory of those final moments would be forever etched on my heart.

It was a new beginning for both of us.

BERNIE'S REFLECTION

Life is not about "why me," but "try me."

Barbara talks throughout her story about faith, hope, and love sustaining her. She also shares her fears. What we must remember is that fear is meant to protect us from dangerous places and things, but it can also deplete our body's resistance to disease and make a situation harder to deal with.

As Barbara drove the car she realized the new role she had taken on. But what she needed to remember was that she and her husband were on the journey together, and the driver doesn't make all the decisions about where they are going. The driver has to ask about and listen to the needs of the passenger even though the driver's experience of the trip may be different. In this case, and in others, the destination is not the driver's choice. You may have considered the question, "How would you live if you knew this was your last day on earth?" But have you ever considered how you would live if it were your loved one's last day? When Barbara drove her husband to the radio station to fulfill his last wish, it became a gift for both of them.

Tears are okay, too. They may make it harder to drive, but they soften the bumps in the road. Trying to eliminate tears and deny feelings is self-destructive and related to denial and depression, not acceptance and finding peace. We are mortal and have feelings, and need to pay attention to them and be guided by them. When we do not pay attention to our needs and feelings, we may develop a lump over our heart as Barbara did.

It is not healthy to deny our needs and care because of what is happening to someone we love. It is more important to do what they would want us to do: to take care of ourselves. Studies show that we are more vulnerable during times of change in our lives, and we can sometimes even predict from therapeutic drawings (when people draw a picture of themselves, their disease, treatment, and immune system) what part of the body will develop a disease during stressful times. This is not about blame, but about our personalities and vulnerabilities due to our internal chemistry during stressful times. So caregivers need to be careful and caring about themselves, too.

Barbara speaks about clarity coming from the awareness of death and the limits of time we have in our lives. We all need to live with that clarity and accept our mortality early on, before we are reminded of it by a diagnosis of a life-threatening illness. Remember, death is not a failure. It is inevitable for us all and for our loved ones. The fact that Dalton could die with his wife by his side tells me that he felt loved and that he knew she was strong enough to survive the loss and begin again.

Dying is not losing the battle. Not experiencing life and love is the real loss. Our lives are about the rhythm we create and not about trying to control the uncontrollable. Your thoughts and attitude are your choice. Barbara worked hard to have the best possible attitude, and it paid off for her.

In any relationship, you never know who is going to die first, so feeling guilty about being the survivor may be something I can understand, but it makes no sense either. For Barbara to feel guilty about enjoying her job is not healthy for her. Life is difficult for all of us, but making other people happy and sacrificing your joy is not how you are supposed to live. Guilt accomplishes nothing unless it changes you for the better through your understanding of why you feel guilty. We all have life issues and challenges; the choice that is available to us is how we face them and what we learn from them. What the experience teaches us is up to us to decide: compassion, hatred, anger, charity. What you do because of your losses is key: your loved one dies and you spend your life hating God and life, or your loved one dies and you start a charity to support others in pain and find a cure for the disease. The choice is yours.

Barbara's story ends with: "It was a new beginning for both of us." Yes, life is a series of beginnings. Every change creates the opportunity for us to begin again.

My Healing Journey

Lynne Zeller

It was a day like so many others, a day in which I was trying to help my son with a high school science project. I was trailing behind him in the craft store as he looked for supplies, and my cell phone rang. "You have mantle cell lymphoma," said the doctor on the other end. Me? I continued my afternoon functioning normally. In fact, I was incredibly calm. On the inside, though, I was in shock and disbelief. Cancer? Not me. I'm healthy; I eat well, I exercise and stay fit, and I'm committed to daily spiritual practice. Other people have cancer, not me. All of a sudden, my ideas of who I was and my sense of control over life were shattered. This was not fair!

I soon discovered that the cancer had spread, not only throughout my lymph system, but also into my spleen and my bone marrow. The prognosis was not great, and my chances of dying from this were very real. My experience of the following weeks was surreal. I was detached from my body and the "normal" world around me, vacillating between feeling numb and disconnected from any emotion, and feeling raw and weepy. How could I tell anyone around me what was happening, especially my family? My concern was that I would have to take care of not only my pain and fear, but theirs too.

At the same time, as a student of Religious Science, I had been taught to view all disease as a wake-up call, to remember our inherent wholeness and perfection, and to let go of false beliefs in separation from our good. I was beginning the second year of an intense two-year training program at my church to become a licensed practitioner. I could see that this was an opportunity to take what had been just abstract concepts before, deep into the core of my being. The way I viewed my cancer shifted from fear and resistance to hope, trust, and expectancy of good.

I brought that same view into the classroom, telling my classmates not long after starting chemo that "I wouldn't trade this experience for anything. It has catapulted me into a new level of experiencing life. I feel so alive and present. I see so many gifts that wouldn't have happened without the cancer. I am confident that this is all divinely guided, that I'm in this experience to learn."

Today I feel just as strongly that cancer was a gift in my life. Deepak Chopra, a physician and a teacher of meditation and therapeutic lifestyle changes, defined health as "the state of perfect physical, mental, social and spiritual well-being" where spiritual well-being is "a state in which a person feels at every moment of living a joy and zest for life, a sense of fulfillment and an awareness of harmony with the universe around him." I am experiencing this well-being in a way I did not know was possible before experiencing cancer.

I've summarized eight practices that have supported me in moving into this wonderfully expanded experience of life, in the hope that they will help others:

1. *Reaching out for support.* A friend of mine warned, "Lynne, do not do cancer the way I did it." She'd told few people about her cancer, went to all of her chemotherapy and radiation sessions by herself, and relied only on her husband for anything she couldn't manage on her own. They were both exhausted and emotionally drained by the experience.

I had always been the strong, giving type and was uncomfortable receiving help, let alone asking for it. But I took her advice to heart. My husband went with me to all of my doctor's appointments. I had friends and family members sit with me for the four-and-a-half-hour chemo sessions. I thought of ways people could help—a friend helped me clean my house, while my family bought me hats and friends quilted with me.

I also paid attention to the many ways people showed they cared. What I learned in this process of asking for and receiving support was how deeply connected we are. Not only did I receive support, I also found that it is a gift to others to gratefully receive.

2. *Choosing to stay present in this moment.* When my doctors told me that this cancer is resistant to treatment and it will recur, my life suddenly felt very precious. Practicing mindfulness in each moment took on more significance for me. I really saw what it meant to be an impartial witness to my experience. Judging things as good or bad would just take me on a roller coaster of emotions that wouldn't aid my healing. By practicing mindfulness before, during, and after the procedures, the pain of my bone marrow biopsies stayed within a short window of time. Mindfulness also means embracing uncertainty in every moment. I realized that everything, not just my medical condition, was ripe with possibility in every moment.

3. *Choosing an attitude of gratitude.* From my hours in the treatment center, a few people stand out in my mind. I remember one woman who was in her eighties. Besides having uterine cancer, she had recently lost her husband and was adjusting to a move. Yet, in talking to her, she seemed so alive and positive; I just wanted to be near her. She wasn't waiting until things got better to live her life.

I've always been an optimistic person. I believe this attitude of seeing the glass as half-full instead of half-empty was a vital part of my healing and of those people I so admired in the treatment center. I believe that we can always find things to be thankful for, and our body responds to this positive outlook. I was grateful to be alive, to spend time with family and friends, to get some exercise, and for some sleep when it came.

I remember I'd often be in tears from the depth of love I felt. I worried less about what people thought of me; instead I let people know how much I loved them.

4. *Holding firm to my dreams.* I am so grateful that I read Larry LeShan's *Cancer as a Turning Point* early in my experience of cancer. I kept reminding myself that if 50 percent of Larry's patients who had been given no hope of survival went into long-term remission, I could certainly regain my health. I need only bring my dreams to life with passion and zeal.

Another person who helped me stay focused on my intentions was Terry McBride. Terry wrote a book called *The Hell I Can't* after enduring a hellish nightmare with *E. coli* over a period of eleven years. What I learned from Terry is that there are dedicated people out there ready to convince you of your limitations. After a while, doubt sets in; perhaps God has a bigger plan for me, perhaps I'm not meant to be healed in my body, perhaps I'll have to go through even more treatment. After talking with Terry, I created a new intention. I took time every day to focus on this intention, actually creating in my mind the experience of being cancer-free, of feeling vitality, well-being, joy, and ease. Whenever fearful thoughts came up, I'd remind myself of these two men and refocus on my intention.

This served me well in June 2003, when I had a consultation with a well-respected lymphoma expert. He was blunt about my poor prognosis. I told myself that I wasn't relying on the medical model for healing and that I was not a statistic. As he spoke, I kept repeating in my mind, "This is not my truth, this is not my truth."

5. *Trusting in a universe that is in a conspiracy for my good.* I believe that we do not live in a random universe. As spiritual beings having a human experience, we have a purpose on earth to wake up to the perfection that we already are.

Everything we encounter in our lives is purposeful and is our unique pathway into the experience of our inherent wholeness. We are like beautiful jewels that have been so crusted over with dirt and grime, we think of ourselves as less-than or lacking. I viewed cancer as a heavy-duty solvent that could support me in experiencing my true, brilliant nature.

I chose to lean into my experience, just as, if I were to fall overboard, I would lean into water, letting it lift me up. I paid attention to whatever I felt myself resisting. For example, one day while getting my chemo infusion, a woman next to me was talking about how she couldn't stand it anymore and wanted to die. I watched myself pulling away from her, wanting to block out the negativity. Only later was I able to see how she triggered my own fears. With that realization, I could embrace the parts in me that didn't want this experience either, and to hold both of us in compassion.

6. *Treating myself as the beloved being that I am.* I had been aware of my pattern of compulsive busyness as an attempt to prove to myself and others that I was okay. However, that didn't stop me from driving myself, judging my performance every step of the way. I wish I could say that my cancer wake-up call immediately cured me of that behavior, but it didn't. Now I have the opportunity to judge the way I did cancer.

A couple of months into my treatment, I described in my journal the experience of jogging with my sister. I was feeling tired and nauseous. I realized that I still had an image of how I should be moving powerfully through treatment. By resisting my experience of exhaustion, of discomfort, I was actually creating more suffering.

The shift was gradual and hard to pinpoint. However, I'm much gentler with myself today and less worried about pleasing other people. I'm saying no more often to those activities that fill my day but don't feed my soul. That judgmental voice in my head is less active today, and I usually remember that it is not who I am.

7. *Connecting with my inner source of intuition.* Cancer treatment can be such an overwhelming experience of decision-making. I've been an alternative health care user for years. My natural health practitioner felt we could successfully treat the lymphoma without chemotherapy. Yet, conversations with my oncologist didn't support her optimism. I am grateful that I had been meditating for years and often turned within for guidance. My inner guidance led me to follow through with my oncologist's recommendation of CHOP chemotherapy in combination with the monoclonal antibody treatment Rituxan, spaced three weeks apart. Throughout this time, I also relied on complementary therapies such as energy work, body work, spiritual guidance, and nutritional changes and supplements to promote my healing. After the sixth session of chemotherapy, the consulting oncologist recommended two more sessions and stem cell harvesting. My intuition led me to stop. I did follow up with two more sessions of Rituxan over the next year. I am so grateful that I could turn to the guidance of a higher source of wisdom throughout my care.

8. *Paying it forward.* I believe that we are all connected. Part of our healing journey is reaching out in our unique way to make this world a better place for others. I have used my own experience with cancer to develop an eight-week class called Revealing Wholeness through Physical Challenge. In addition to teaching this class, I facilitate a couple of support groups and counsel individuals. This work feeds my soul and keeps the lessons fresh in my life as I support others on their healing journeys.

When I turned fifty in 2002, I thought my life was good. Little could I imagine the fullness, the joy, the loving connection to others and the sense of purposefulness that cancer, of all things, would bring into my life later that year. It was three and a half years before I had a recurrence—much longer than the doctors expected. I am confident that these eight practices made a difference. A new drug treatment, Velcade, helped bring me back into remission. My life is so much bigger now than it was as I stood in the aisle of the craft store that day. Just as my son has moved beyond high school science projects and into a college world of greater freedom and possibility, I, too, have moved into a much richer world.

BERNIE'S REFLECTION

There are many side effects to accepting your mortality,
and they're not all bad.

Lynne Zeller has said it all. To express the wisdom she expressed in this story, most people would need to write a book. Her wisdom did not come easily, however. It came from experiencing a disaster. She doesn't sound like a survivor at the beginning of her journey. She begins by expressing how she lost her sense of control and how she did not share with her family because she didn't want to upset them and have to deal with their feelings. That is far from survival behavior. If you are facing a life-threatening illness, and focusing on what you can't control and how to not upset your family, you are in big trouble.

But as the story moved on, Lynne underwent a transformation or rebirth. Remember, no one can change you. You have to be willing to learn how to change, to become responsible and participate in your change. Religious Science is a great teacher, and I have always loved the work of its founder, Ernest Holmes. Lynne combined all of her resources in order to heal, and with that came a momentous shift. She was no longer a victim who was not in control. She realized her thoughts and actions are what she could control, and that made all the difference in her perspective of her disease.

Because of what cancer taught her about life, Lynne came to view it as a gift. I am sure she would like to be completely cured of her gift, but she would not give up the education it provided her. I disagree, in a way, with Deepak Chopra's comment about health being about perfection. I see many people who are in good health and who have incurable diseases. They are still very much alive and see their lives as gifts, too. I think Helen Keller was one of the healthiest people ever, but her body wasn't perfect. I could cite many more examples, people like Max Cleland, who lost his legs and an arm when a hand grenade exploded but has served in the U.S. Senate and is a healed man. His autobiography is entitled *Strong at the Broken Places*. Health is about attitude and your state of mind more than it is about your body.

Lynne's list offers concrete tools to stimulate survival behavior and enhance immune-competent personality characteristics. I believe it would benefit patients greatly if doctors would share such a list with their patients. Lynne speaks of reaching out to others, and this is supported by studies that reveal we experience less pain when we are accompanied to the hospital by a loved one, whether it is a child being inoculated or an adult receiving chemotherapy. Living in the moment is another important point Lynne awakens to. When you live in the moment, you are actually creating the future in a much more positive way than worrying about it would do.

Being grateful also makes an enormous difference. What others think of you is what occupies many people's minds. In Lynne's case, having cancer gave her the courage to be able to stop worrying about what other people thought of her.

Lynne practiced meditation to tap into her intuition and use it for guidance and direction. Another method I have found is to pay attention to your dreams and drawings. Your inner wisdom— call it intuition if you will—and your body can speak to you through many modalities. Not enough is taught about this in medical school. Lynne speaks of her desire and the difference it made in her life. Also, doctors don't often emphasize how important attitude and intention can be in the healing process.

I remember my friend Larry LeShan, whom Lynne mentions, writing about a gang leader with life-threatening cancer who had lost all interest in living because of his illness and inability to be involved in a gang. Larry got him a job in the fire department, which provided the same environment of camaraderie and danger as his gang. His cancer went into remission and he became well.

He called Larry years later, worried because they wanted to promote him to an office job and he was concerned his cancer might come back in that environment. We always need to stay aware of what feeds our soul as well.

There is intelligence and survival behavior in nature, but we have much more complicated lives that require work in order to achieve the state of mind and healing that we are naturally capable of. Most so-called miracles are not accidents. They begin to happen when we do what Lynne did. She started to say no! That is the most important thing you can do with your life's time. Use it in the way you decide and not the way imposed by others' requests.

In closing, let me say that if you don't die from your disease in the time you were originally given in your prognosis, please note as Lynne did that other treatments become available. So technology and science are to be acknowledged for their gifts, too.

Remember, as Lynne did, to keep beginning. There is no end to the number of transformations, rebirths, and healings you can achieve and experience in your life's time.

Baby Jamie: A Survivor's Story

Elaine Ambrose

My brother-in-law, Jim Romano, drove down the freeway toward his home with the simple goal of picking up his two young children from school. But his mind was reeling and he couldn't focus, even though he knew what he had to do at that moment. Tears clouded his eyes as he slammed his hand on the steering wheel and yelled a cry that came from his very core. Finally, unable to drive any further, he pulled over to the side of the road and broke down in uncontrollable sobs. He and his wife had just learned that their thirteen-month-old daughter had leukemia.

So began a two-year ordeal when life would change and would never be the same again for the Romano family. Jim would take on the responsibility of caring for Andrew, then age five, and Michelle, then age four, while he continued his job as a realtor in the Denver, Colorado, area. His wife, Andrea, would focus on baby Jamie and spend most of her time at Children's Hospital in Denver. Ultimately, Jamie's leukemia would become the catalyst that would bring together an extended family and also galvanize a group of volunteers to establish a thriving annual fund-raising program that continues to benefit hundreds of other children with life-threatening illnesses.

The Rocky Mountains were brilliant, as usual, during the fall of 2000. My husband, Michael, and I had joined his brother Jim and his family at their cabin in southern Colorado. We took walks in the woods with their three children, played games at the big wooden table, and prepared hearty meals. I particularly enjoyed holding thirteen-month-old Jamie. She had big blue eyes and a sweet disposition. We all commented on what a contented baby she was and how she liked to be held. My husband noticed that the baby's exotic coloring gave her a Mediterranean look, a true Italian of Romano heritage. Andrea, our sister-in-law, commented that she was taking the baby in for a medical examination the following week.

Little did we know that the docile baby was, in fact, dying. We received the horrific news the following week that Jamie had been diagnosed with leukemia. By then we were back at our home in Idaho and felt helpless and worried. Jamie was scheduled immediately for chemotherapy treatments, and for the first time, we cried and prayed together.

Chemotherapy is brutal, especially for babies. Her soft hair fell out, she suffered from infections, and her tiny veins were prodded daily with needles. Because of her age, she didn't talk, so she couldn't communicate her needs or pains. At times, the doctors were baffled about the exact diagnosis. Then they concluded that Jamie had a rare blood disorder that complicated her treatment. She then suffered through several days of full-body radiation treatments.

As Andrea stayed at the hospital with Jamie, Jim kept working and caring for the other two children. He set up a Web site so concerned family and friends could stay informed about the prognosis. Volunteers from Jim's work and from their church stepped in to provide meals, child care, and comfort. Jim's four adult siblings lived far away, from Alaska to Arkansas, but they rallied around to help. Jim's sister took time from her job and came from Alaska to help with the children and organize the home. When Jamie's treatments became more intense, Jim's sister in Arkansas offered to keep Andrew and

Michelle at her home. Jim left his wife and baby at the hospital, flew the other two children to Arkansas, and returned to his job. He went to the hospital each night after work and then spent his evenings alone, organizing insurance papers and updating the Web site.

After several months, the family was reunited at home. Andrea took medical training to care for Jamie, which included giving her shots into a port attached to the baby's chest. The other two children accepted their new reality. The house had to be professionally cleaned and quarantined. No friends could come over and play. Jamie had to wear a mask, and everyone had to be careful not to disturb the bandage over her chest. In remarkable fashion, Jamie rarely cried, and she sat patiently as her mother gave her shots and medication. She seemed to know what she had to do in order to live.

My husband and I visited several times during Jamie's ordeal. Michael loves to cook, so he made some authentic Italian meals for the family. I was the "sous chef," and we created several recipes that could be frozen for a later time. I enjoyed playing with the two older children as Andrea took care of Jamie. Michael and his brother Jim often retreated to the patio after dinner for a soothing glass (or four) of wine. We all discovered that the trauma of Jamie's illness was bringing the family together more than ever before.

Jamie continued to have problems with recovery. At one point, the doctor talked to Jim and Andrea about a bone marrow transfusion. They were tested, but didn't match. So Jim sat down with his two children and talked about how they could help save their sister. The young boy and girl volunteered to be tested and, like strong soldiers, went to the hospital to have their blood drawn. Unfortunately, they were not a match. It became an ordeal of hospital visits, more procedures, and different medications. One medication caused hair to grow on Jamie's back. Jim joked that he'd gladly take a hairy daughter because she was still alive.

Finally, Jamie was scheduled for a bone marrow transplant. The procedure involved taking stem cells from the umbilical cord of a healthy newborn baby. The stem cells were injected into Jamie and she had a complete bone marrow transfusion. Jim and Andrea brought Andrew and Michelle to the hospital to see their little sister. In the Oncology and Bone Marrow Transplant Ward of Children's Hospital, she was hooked to tubes and machines, but they were allowed to wear masks and touch her and read her a story. Their tenderness brought tears to the eyes of attending nurses.

After a year of treatments and hospital stays, Jamie finally came home for an extended time. Jim's and Andrea's parents all lived in the Denver area and were eager to help however they could. Jamie began to improve as Andrea continued her care. She learned to crawl and started speaking a few words. Her physical and mental development had been delayed by the chemotherapy and radiation, but she started to make up for lost time. Andrea remembered with joy the first time she carried Jamie outside without her mask. The entire family climbed up on the fort in the backyard, ate watermelon, and spit out the seeds. Jamie was, indeed, their miracle baby.

To celebrate the life of their baby girl and to help other families in need, the Romano family felt compelled to organize a fund-raising event. Starting a charity program is a daunting task, so Jim brought together a group of loyal coworkers and committed friends to investigate the possibility of starting a foundation. They did research on the Internet on how to set up a program, they obtained pro bono legal advice, and they talked with other foundations and charities in the Denver area. They studied local, regional, and national non-profit materials and reviewed grant information. Finally, they met with event planners to learn how to coordinate the best venue to launch their program. Throughout the complicated process, the initial group found strength and inspiration as they focused on their benevolent goals.

In 2001 Jim and his company established the Prestige Miracles Foundation. They enlisted volunteers to organize a walk and run event called Miracles for Miles as a fund-raiser to provide assistance to other children and families in the Denver metro area. Their first event was attended by a few hundred people and raised around $10,000 for Children's Hospital. Today the mission of the foundation has evolved to include multiple events and additional categories of recipients. The foundation's mission is to improve the lives of children diagnosed with life-threatening illness, or those who are faced with a lifetime medical condition, or those who are involved in tragic accidents. Over the years, the foundation has raised and donated almost one million dollars for charity.

The foundation sponsors three main events. Miles for Miracles is a 5K and Family Fun Run, and participants can register online or at participating sponsors. The day concludes with awards, several drawings, and entertainment. Prizes are awarded according to age group, from under twelve to over seventy, and DJ music is provided by Robert Romano, Jim's brother. At one event, I watched baby Jamie so her parents and siblings could participate in the race. The entire family crossed the finish line with smiles and feelings of achievement and gratitude. Proceeds from the race are donated to the Children's Hospital and to other children in need.

The second event, Birdies for Blessings, is a golf tournament that features many well-known Denver companies as sponsors. The popular event raises money through tournament fees, dinner, and a silent auction. Jim golfs in the event with his son, Andrew, and other family members participate as needed. Michael and I golf in the event and provide sponsorship through our publishing company. Michael loves to have me on his team because my high handicap helps us win. It amazes me that my incompetence actually turns out to be an asset!

Cheers for Charities is the third event, and it's very popular for those who would rather sip wine than jog or golf. The wine-tasting soiree raises funds to provide modest financial grants to needy children and their families. Grants are limited to $2,000 and are used to provide short-term assistance to allow the family to stay in their home or to pay for special furnishings or technologies. Recipients have received such gifts as a pump for a girl with diabetes and Christmas gifts for the seven children of a woman suffering from Lou Gehrig's disease. Some grants are given to promote research in the name of a child who has died from cancer. Additional information and online grant applications are found at www.milesformiracles.com.

Every birthday is another miracle for Jamie Romano. Because of the intense radiation treatments at such a young age, she is small for her age. The procedures impacted the quality of her teeth and her organs, and she'll be on medications for the rest of her life. But that doesn't stop her from being a beautiful, active, and smart young girl. She keeps up with her older brother and sister, and she's a tough competitor on her soccer team. She's full of mischief, and she's also full of life.

Many years ago I held Jamie as a lethargic, sick baby. Now she touches my heart with a special connection that carries a profound message of strength and survival. Sometimes she looks far away and seems to communicate with spiritual powers. We remain in awe of her ability to bring our family together from the depths of despair. With faith, hope, modern medical technology, and a charitable foundation, Jamie continues to spread joy to her family and throughout her community.

BERNIE'S REFLECTION

Every life is a marathon, and the goal is to finish yours.

As a medical student and pediatric surgeon, I used to wonder why God would create a world where innocent children would suffer from cancer and other problems. It was never discussed as part of medical training. It took me a long time, and some conversations with God, to understand that a perfect world is not creation. It is a magic trick. What makes this a meaningful world is that people have choices, and when love is demonstrated it means something. So we are all here to live and learn. There are no mistakes, just lessons to be learned. I think what Jamie's parents did was to learn from their heartbreak and create a better world through their love and compassion.

Life never stops changing. It is about beginnings, just as the graduation ceremony celebrating the end of your schooling is called a commencement and not a termination. To start to raise funds and benefit others is what life is ultimately about. A new beginning and a new life come from compassion. A young man I knew well named Toni Fenton, when dying due to cystic fibrosis, asked me, "Why am I different?" He wanted to know why he was dying when other teenagers were out playing in the street. I answered him from someplace deep within me, "Toni, because it makes you beautiful." I was about to apologize when he looked up with a beautiful smile and understood. In his name millions of dollars have been raised to help other children with his disease. He touched everyone who knew him and is immortal through his love.

When you are motivated by your affliction, you can create change in the world through participating in such things as volunteering, charities, support groups, and more. The pain of being a doctor changed my life and made me want to help people live and not just treat their diseases. A friend of mine, Roxanne, has lupus. She started the Friends Health Connection to bring people together and support one another. I asked her once how she got so many important people to speak for her organization in New Jersey, including Deepak Chopra, Andy Weil, and Rabbi Kushner. Her answer: "I drive them crazy." Her wounds motivate her and they make her very special, too.

Years ago my phone rang and when I answered a man said, "My son has leukemia and I want you to join us and run in the New York marathon to raise funds for lymphoma and leukemia research." My reaction was that you had to be crazy to do that, but I did it because he wouldn't take no for an answer. That was in 1988 and the organization he started hasn't stopped growing since that first event. And yes, I have run several marathons and think that every life is a marathon and the goal is to finish yours. I will never forget a woman standing on the curb in Manhattan who said as we passed, "You're all winners."

I am sure Jamie had less trouble with her disease—and has less trouble even now with her limitations—than her parents did. Children and animals are great teachers who live in the moment and can accept their bodies and their problems and still keep loving. People like Jamie and her family are not disabled, they are enabled.

Learning to Let Go

Cindy Hurn

My first introduction to cancer came unexpectedly when I was eight years old. Our mother went into the hospital for an operation, and kindly neighbors invited my older sister and me to their house for supper. Sitting at the dining room table, I happily aimed a forkful of delicious food into my mouth. As I chewed, I overheard Florence in the kitchen whisper to her husband, "Whatever will those girls do if their mother dies?" Suddenly the piece of food grew; the pressure of it filled my mouth, throat, head, ears, and eyes. . . . I couldn't swallow. I couldn't see. I couldn't hear. I couldn't breathe. I desperately tried to conceal my panic, masking calmness so that no one would discover I had overheard the whispered and private conversation. I was afraid—no, terrified—of knowing something that I shouldn't. Adults had such strange rules, and through my innocent curiosity, I frequently discovered that I had broken them.

The memory of that day was vividly branded upon the core of my child-brain. It was a moment of paralyzing fear—the threat of my mother's death, my inability to breathe, and the sudden perception that I, too, might die. I realize now that if I had just opened my mouth and released the food, I could have cried out and been comforted—but children don't know these things, so I held back my tears and hid my fears deep in the tissues of my belly.

Our father finally gave us the news—our mother had terminal cancer, and the doctors said she had six months to live. Mom wanted to be at home, not in a hospital. Dad asked us girls, only nine and ten years old, if we would be prepared to take care of our mother until she died. We could, and we would.

Reaching for other hope, my dad went to an oncologist at Yale-New Haven Hospital. Not only did he agreed to see my mother, but when he read through her notes and finished examining her, he said, "I can't tell you how long you are going to live any more than I can predict my own life span, but I can tell you this: In six months from now, you will not be dead. In six months you will be dancing again."

How I wish I could speak to that doctor now and thank him for the encouragement and commitment that he and his team gave to my family. The doctor kept his promise. Six months later, Dad brought Mom to New York City—and they danced at their favorite swing band dance hall. I remember getting goose bumps of excitement when Mom paraded out in front of us in her new dress and shoes, minutes before they left for the dance. She looked so happy, so full of life! That night meant the world to my parents. It was the last time they danced. Days later, Mom's femur bone broke and the pattern of operations, hospital treatments, and recovery returned to our lives.

My mother lived for three more years. Some days were good. We lived as normal a life as possible, and during that period we treasured the times that Mom could share with us. In my school talent show I played my guitar and sang, and Mom sat in her wheelchair in the front row with tears of pride wetting her face. We made summer visits to Cape Cod, where we swam in the bay, calling out, "Watch me swim, Mommy—watch me!" And she watched and smiled and told us how proud she was of her girls.

We have many memories of Mom today because of the inspired doctor who challenged our mother's appointed death. The doctor ordered her new treatments and medicine, but most importantly, fed her large doses of confidence and hope. He encouraged her and gave her permission to live as long as she could for her girls. I think of him as a very special angel in my life.

The difficult times taught my sister and me many things. We learned about resolve, faith, persistence, and love. My sister chose to enter the nursing field, and over the years she has saved many lives and helped countless patients and families to cope with illness and the healing process. I raised money each year for cancer research, and in middle age became a long-term volunteer in an international breast cancer research trial. The decision to join as a healthy test subject was easy, and the involvement was empowering for me.

From my earliest memories, cancer had been a hungry monster that devoured the people I loved. My mother was only one of many family members who succumbed to the awful disease. In a strange and sick sort of way, I felt like I would have to get the disease in order to fight the beast and win. By being part of an international study, one that was making great strides in breast cancer detection and prevention, I no longer needed to make my body a battleground. From then on, I determined that "Besieged by Cancer" was not going to be my story, and to this day I have been blessed with cancer-free health.

Over the years I have met many women who experienced the disease. What impressed me, time and time again, was that the women who felt loved and valued, and who had a focused purpose in their lives, were the ones who either survived, or died more peacefully. With new drug treatments and procedures, more and more people live to say that the experience of cancer changed their lives for the better. The word "cancer" used to draw gasps and looks of horror from people. But as have years passed and medical knowledge has gained momentum, the word "cancer" has lost much of its daunting power. The motherless child in me triumphantly gloats each time I see the monster shrinking.

Six years ago I was unexpectedly reunited with my first love, Rich, my childhood sweetheart. We had lost touch with each other soon after he went to Vietnam, and by the time he returned, I had moved to another country. Thirty-four years later, we accidentally discovered each other on the Internet. Tentatively at first, we exchanged stories of our lives, and before long, daily e-mails crossed the miles between England and the United States.

I previously had planned to return to the United States after my daughter's wedding, and settle in the Northwest. When our cyberspace relationship grew, I told my "old flame" of the plans and arranged to visit him for a few days before heading up to the Northwest. He'd gone through the heartbreak of a broken marriage four years before, and now lived alone and worked at his accountancy business while putting his kids through college.

We realized that the likelihood of falling in love when we met in person was quite small. Through electronic letters and long-distance calls, we ignited the dreams of our youth. But the reality of middle-aged bodies and settled personalities was more likely to leave us feeling estranged or disappointed. We decided to take things slowly, to enjoy a short reunion. Perhaps, after I settled up north, we might get together from time to time. If we were lucky, a second chance at finding love might eventually transpire.

Soon after I arrived at Rich's house, I could see that he was not a well man. He told me that shortly after his marriage ended, a mole on his leg began to fester. He was diagnosed with melanoma and had been receiving treatment for a few years. A recent checkup revealed one growth that had gone frighteningly deep. When we met, he was just recovering from surgery and drug treatment. The news floored me. That damned cancer was back in my life again! I finally had a chance to open my heart and look toward a love-filled future, but now it seemed that Rich, too, was going to be taken away.

After a few days I realized that Rich might need help in his office while he recovered his strength and energy. After all, he was an accountant and I was a bookkeeper. Maybe I had been brought back into his life to help him during this difficult time. I had no job to lose or responsibilities that would suffer in my absence. I decided then to stay for a few weeks and put my Northwest plans back until Christmas.

During the next two months our old relationship seemed to take up just where it left off, though with a softer maturity.

I began to take care of my friend in such a way that he knew he was needed and knew he was loved. I gave him frequent massages, cooked healthy foods, and packed him healthy lunches. Though he complained with gusto about the amount of "green stuff" in his new diet, he ate the meals I prepared, knowing they contained the elements of health and healing. For the first time in years, he had someone special in his life, someone who actively cared about him. We worked together, laughed together, loved together. As our love grew and deepened, my friend's health and vitality returned.

Christmas came and went. By now we felt that we were meant to be together again. The second-chance relationship that each of us dreamt about was unfolding and filling our days with new hope. It was then that I decided to stay.

All was not rosy, however. I had trouble accepting his method of dealing with his cancer. He seemed to take it almost nonchalantly. Once, during tax season, he canceled an appointment with the dermatologist, saying he was too busy! I nearly went nuts trying to convince him to go to the doctor; join this trial; try that food; ask about other treatments, and so on. He nearly went nuts putting up with my panic!

I was an emotional wreck. One day I fled to a friend's house in tears. She sat me down in her kitchen with a mug of coffee as I poured out my feelings of both heartache and the frustration I felt from trying to make my partner take his disease seriously. I expected sympathy and understanding. Much to my surprise, she told me that it was not my disease to worry about. She explained that my behavior was intrusive, self-seeking, and that it showed disrespect for my partner's ability to handle the disease in his own way. "In fact," she said, "I think you owe him an apology."

I suddenly realized how right she was. I went back and apologized to Rich, promising that I would stop trying to control his cancer and that he could have it all to himself. Instead, I would enjoy taking care of him, loving him, and playing golf with him! If he wanted to discuss it with me, I would listen, but I would no longer badger him with questions and expectations. And I stuck to my promise. For a long time, he wouldn't say anything to me about the condition. Some days he would come home with Band-Aids on his body or a few stitches. I would breathe a private sigh of relief, knowing he had been to the doctor and received treatment. After a couple of years of keeping my promise, Rich felt comfortable enough to bring the subject up and talk about his worries or ask me to check a mole on his back or his scalp.

Now, when my heart cringes with the fear of losing him, I discuss those feelings with my women friends. The change in my attitude and behavior created a healthy boundary of mutual trust and respect with my sweetheart. We adopted the habit of living each day as it comes and filling that day with the best we could give it. We don't worry about tomorrow; we challenge each other to get that hole-in-one on our favorite golf course; we do the grocery shopping together, listen to records, and, like my own parents once did, dance to the slow music of our teens.

Instead of grieving about what cancer has taken from my life, I now experience joy from what cancer put into it. Compassion. Patience. Learning to love each person as a perfect being within the imperfections of human existence. I learned not to fear; to know that life unfolds just as it is meant to. By showing me how to love better, cancer filled my life with purpose and gently prodded me to sit amid the gratitude of life's many blessings.

BERNIE'S REFLECTION

Seek peace, because when you wage a war against cancer,
you empower your enemy.

Cindy acknowledges what we all experience in our early years: that children are often hypnotized by what they hear from various authority figures. She writes the words "vividly branded upon the core of my child-brain." When fear and death are embedded in a child's brain, imagine what that does to her life. We all need to deal with the negative and destructive messages that are embedded in our consciousness in a therapeutic and healing way.

She didn't cry out for help. That I believe is related not just to her age, but also to family patterns and messages. We need to be comfortable making noise, crying out, being angry, and getting attention when we need it. Animals do not worry about what you are thinking when they make noise, move, and display emotion to gain your attention, and we must understand that this is survival behavior.

Cindy says she hid fears deep in the tissues of her belly. When she did that, she set herself up for possible future diseases. When we focus negative energy and fear upon parts of our body, we make those parts more susceptible to illness. Some people even hate their bodies and see them as a threat. Love your body, just as it loves you, and remember to give it love messages, not fear messages.

Then something nice happened to Cindy: in walked Doctor Hope. What has frustrated me for decades is that doctors do not receive training about how to care for people and not just treat their disease. Doctors keep their power by predicting when their patients will die. They often experience change when they, or their families, are suddenly the patients. I know of many wonderful stories told by doctors who learned to give their loved ones hope and how it affected their survival.

One very important lesson Cindy learned was to not see cancer as the enemy and to not wage a continuous battle that would take over her life. She says, "I felt like I would have to get the disease in order to fight the beast and win." She evolves and finishes with, "I no longer needed to make my body a battleground. "Yes! What we need to do is make our lives and bodies places of healing and not war. We need to find inner peace.

At the same time, Cindy sensed the qualities that survivors need: love, value, and meaning in their lives. You also have to follow the advice I am constantly sharing: do what will make you happy. Finding Rich and staying with him felt right. That's the reason to do something—when it feels right and not because you think you should do it.

You have to let go of others and, as with Rich, give them their disease. Why he doesn't do what is best for him is his issue. It can be to get attention or because he doesn't love himself as much as Cindy loves him. The reason is not important. What one must do is love him until he loves and cares about himself enough to act that way.

In the end, Cindy has learned to share her feelings with friends and live for today, and that the side effects of cancer are not all bad. These include freedom from fear and to love better. So there are gifts in every experience, and when you are a survivor you will open yourself to them and experience a new life free of the fears of the past.

What We Could Do Together

Connie Curley

W hat kind of a marriage is this?" I thought, putting down the phone after talking to my husband. "Should I leave?"

At the time, it seemed to me I was living my own version of the biblical story of Job. First both my parents passed away. Then my husband, Paul, was transferred halfway across the country to the state of Washington. This unexpected company move brought on yet another tribulation—selling our home. Paul had left already for the West Coast. I stayed behind with our two teenage children in Illinois, hoping someone, anyone, would make a bid on our place.

But who would buy it? The area where we were living was experiencing an economic depression, and our place was quite large and more than a little unusual. It was the only California ranch style residence in that small Midwestern town, which was essentially Victorian—architecturally, politically, and spiritually. Once I put the house on the market, everyone wanted to see what it was like inside, but no one wanted to buy it.

Using the newest and best of everything, our home had been built by a highly skilled contractor for his own family. The exterior was constructed of stone. Inside, the four-inch-thick concrete floors were supported every two feet by steel I beams. The house measured 3,200 square feet aboveground and 3,800 square feet below. We are convinced the contractor had been thinking "bomb shelter" when he built it. Although we liked the place, it was not everyone's idea of a home. I tried all the tricks of the trade, from newspaper ads and open houses to repainting and documenting the efficiency of the insulation by publishing our heating bills.

The two long years it took for the house to sell were bleak. Paul's visits home became less frequent, and as the months passed he seemed to become oblivious to our lives in Illinois. During one phone call, I explained to him, "The poor old Volvo is having some alternator problems. The mechanic at the service station on Main Street says he thinks he can take care of it, though." It was a small but sturdy two-door 1976 model with a sunroof. It had always been dependable, and it was fun to drive. I didn't want to trade it in. Two weeks after that conversation, I again mentioned the alternator problems. "Oh," he said, "I didn't know you were having any trouble with the car." Some helpmate he was.

As I packed boxes and cartons for my long-awaited move to Washington, my husband felt it was time to warn me what life would be like after I'd settled. "You need to know I will most likely be traveling even more now with a new sales territory."

Wonderful. All I could think was, "What kind of marriage is this? Our son is staying behind in Illinois, while our daughter is going off to college. We've been living two thousand miles apart for most of the last two years. And now, after working so hard to sell the house and to be together under one roof, I'm going to be left home, alone?" Well, that was it. If what he had said became reality, I decided silently, I would leave my marriage. What had once been a loving partnership seemed to be ending.

Ten short days after moving into the new home in Washington, Paul answered his business phone. "I thought you'd give me more time," I heard him say sadly. Just like that, his sales job had dissolved.

The next couple of days we were numbed by what had happened. I have to admit, though, I was relieved Paul wouldn't be traveling. At least we were together. We slowly started functioning again as a partnership, brainstorming on how to attack the situation. I arranged to begin the paperwork for obtaining a Washington teacher's certificate. Looking for almost any place that might be able to use me, I contacted a local community college where one phone call led to another, and I was offered a contract to teach two remedial classes on a part-time basis for one quarter. Paul was hired by a small business to write resumes a few hours each week. Things were looking up. We were acting more like a couple, and the healing of our marriage had begun.

Since I hadn't had a physical exam in quite a while, I decided to have one in the limited time we had remaining with the health insurance from Paul's former company. One afternoon shortly after school started, I headed to the gynecologist expecting to be told, as usual, "Everything seems fine. I'll see you in a year." No, instead I heard, "I would like to see you again in a month." Four weeks later she repeated the same words. When I saw her the third time, her comments were different, and her voice was clipped and business-like. "See the person at the front desk to set up an appointment for surgery. Your right ovary might have to be removed."

Two weeks later an unfamiliar doctor entered my hospital room and seated himself on a chair near the bed. "You have ovarian cancer." The oncologist's words were blunt as he spoke to Paul and me. I wasn't surprised by the diagnosis. Earlier in the week, my optimistic physician had told me the mass was probably just a nonmalignant tumor, requiring only an hour and a half in the operating room. The procedure had begun at 8:00 A.M. on the Tuesday before Thanksgiving 1984. The moment I awoke from the anesthesia, I saw the clock on the wall: 2:30 P.M. I knew.

Still somewhat under the effects of medication that following day, I felt detached as the doctor continued talking. "We have our work cut out for us. You have a fifty-fifty chance of living for one year. Because you are young and your veins are good, we're going to hit you hard with the chemotherapy. We'll start in one month." He offered no comforting words. As ridiculous as it sounds, my thoughts quickly ran to the cruise Paul and I had dreamed for years of doing "sometime." We might never be able to do it!

"What are we going to do?" I asked when the doctor had left the room. "I don't think I will be able to continue working while undergoing chemotherapy. How will we survive?" The resume-writing job had proven to be financially useless, and Paul had not been able to find any lucrative work. My meager salary as a part-time instructor was our only source of income for the time being. While I was contemplating what I couldn't do, my husband was considering what we could do together. He devised a plan.

Because the disease had spread to some lymph nodes, the cocktail of chemicals that the doctor intended to use would include Cisplatin, the administration of which required that I be in the hospital for a minimum of thirty-six hours once each month during the eight months of treatment.

Paul suggested we do a trial run of his plan while the school was on winter break. That way, without jeopardizing my classes, we could see if his idea would work. So the Friday before Christmas, I was scheduled for the oncologist's last appointment of the day. When he was satisfied with the results from the blood tests, he informed the hospital I would check in by 8:00 P.M. Knowing the chemotherapy might make me nauseated, Paul took me out for a nice dinner—a kind of "last meal."

We watched TV in my hospital room until he went home shortly after 10:00 P.M. By Saturday morning, despite antinausea medication, I was more than nauseated. Paul returned to my bedside and held my head for most of the day while I vomited. Never mind the time he forgot my Volvo was acting up, this was love.

Sunday morning I was able to eat a little food, and I was permitted to go home at noon. Once there, with Paul's encouragement I ate a bit of chicken noodle soup and nibbled on crackers between naps. By Monday afternoon, I was feeling almost like myself. The plan was manageable. The classes I would be teaching on Fridays for the upcoming quarter were scheduled for early in the day. Mondays I had only an evening class. I would not have to quit my job. We were functioning as a team, again.

Thus, every four weeks, Paul's plan became our routine. Additionally, he insisted I take a nap every day while he cooked dinner. By experience, we learned that I could avoid nausea between treatments if I didn't let my stomach get empty, so I snacked frequently. Paul placed oyster crackers and M&M's on my night side table next to the bed so I could have a bite to eat if I wakened before morning. He told me, "Bald is sexy and beautiful." He arranged for a short vacation one weekend. He went to every doctor appointment with me. How could I ever have questioned his devotion?

When my chemotherapy ended, I had what was called "Second Look Surgery." The pathologist's report showed no sign of cancer in any of the thirteen biopsies. Any questions I might have had about God's goodness or faithfulness were dispelled. Yes, the cancer treatments resulted in many negative side effects. My urine turned bright red during the chemotherapy treatments. I experienced a great deal of nausea, and I had days in which I consistently vomited. I lost weight and endeavored to wear clothes that would hide my skeletal frame. I lost all my hair. My blood count went down. My energy level took a dive. But if I had not had to deal with those challenges, I doubt I would have learned the true extent of Paul's love for me and my love for him. In addition to a strengthening of my faith, the wonderful unexpected side effect of all we went through is a truly solid, exceptionally happy marriage that is still strong twenty-three years later. Indeed, God works all things for the good.

BERNIE'S REFLECTION

Invest in your relationships and everyone benefits.

When you are pondering, as Connie was, if you should leave a marriage, there are three possible answers. The first options are that you can separate or get a divorce. However, if the marriage is not threatening your health or life, then ask yourself how love could resolve the problem and how you could then live the answer. Look at the love Connie found later in her marriage and how it has healed her life and Paul's life.

You have to understand that you are not a victim. You have choices, and let your heart participate in the answer. Also, when separated from your loved ones, learn how to listen to each other.

When you do, you will understand each other's experiences and not get upset when, for example, your spouse forgets about the Volvo's alternator. With open communication, you will know where his mind is and what problems he is encountering that make the Volvo insignificant. Whenever you are separated from a loved one, always ask about her feelings and thoughts. Listen to her words without offering solutions, but try to provide compassion and understanding.

After two years of separation from her husband, Connie developed ovarian cancer. The stress coming from her situation could have had a direct impact on her immune system. Years ago I realized the importance of asking my patients what had happened in the last year or two of their lives. We have to realize that our body chemistry and internal messaging are affecting our health, and that what the cells in our body are exposed to affects their behavior. We need to look at more than the physical when treating a disease.

Then Cindy had the noncompassionate message from the oncologist: You have a fifty-fifty chance of surviving a year and we will "hit" you hard with chemotherapy. Why do doctors hit, poison, blast, burn, and assault the body with chemotherapy, radiation, and surgery? Why can't they talk about healing, eliminating, curing, and helping you to survive? Doctors need to learn how to communicate and induce positive side effects and healing. Patients need to feel they can say no if they don't feel right about the doctor or his suggestions or attitude, or when the result of his visit is a negative one.

Finally, let me share the story of a woman who was handed a bag to vomit in by her husband as he was driving her home after chemotherapy. She told me, "I opened the bag and there were a dozen roses from my husband in it. I never vomited again." Connie's symbolic dozen roses arrived in the way her husband showed he cared and loved her. That is what healing is about and why loved ones can make it through hell when their beloved is with them. Her husband was far more than a mechanic and a chauffeur. Don't wait for cancer to bring forth your love and your feelings.

Making My Own Music

Paula Neustadt

I stood ankle-deep in the shallow pool of warm water and stabilized my footing among the slippery rocks, face-to-face with a woman whom I had just met and whose urban demeanor was a frenetic intrusion to the calm and serenity I had just spent hours nurturing for myself.

I had come to these canyon hot springs knowing I would be soothed by the healing waters and the surrounding beauty of nature. There was a strong sense of connection to be found here, a sense of being a part of the universe along with the flowing river; swaying reeds; scent of white, blue, and purple sage; water-shaped rocks; slimy green algae; geothermal bubbles; clear winter sky; low-angled sun; and sloping mountain peak. The ever-changing forces of time and movement were potently evident in everything around me and in me, and I felt a reassurance that all vitality springs forth from change.

The woman had arrived with her two companions as I was about to depart. Before her arrival I had spent a portion of my time cradled and supported by the water's surface tension as I relaxed into a floating posture and allowed my stress and anxiety to sink away. Then I faced the mountain and thought of it as The Mountain found in many cultures' creation stories, referred to as The Place of their origins. I had come to this place to prepare myself for my upcoming breast cancer surgery on December 23.

Years before, while suffering from depleted emotional and physical energy, I visited an ashram and experienced the value that chanting had in enhancing my stamina, strength, and clarity. I wanted to be in the most optimum condition I could be in before my surgery, and I knew chanting would be one of my avenues in that direction. There in that peaceful setting, alone in the wilderness, I repeated the verses again and again until I no longer chanted the chant but the chant chanted me, a state also known as "the flow."

> May the blessings of God rest upon you,
> May God's peace abide with you,
> May God's presence illuminate your heart,
> Now and forever more
>
> Oh Grandmother come to me,
> Heal my spirit, mind and body.
>
> The Earth, she is my mother,
> I will take care of her.
>
> Listen, listen, listen to my heart-song.
> I will never forsake you.
> I will always love you.
>
> Earth my body, water my blood,
> Air my breath and fire my spirit.

After chanting alone at the hot springs I planned to again visit the ashram, where I intended to be infused with the Sanskrit chants from a sanctuary full of Vedantic devotees. But suddenly my plans were halted when this intrusive stranger asked for my help and instruction in chanting, and here I stood about to begin to teach her.

Could I teach someone to chant? I doubted my own knowledge, being more experienced at being a seeker than a teacher. But as she pleaded, I realized that indeed I could teach her one that I had just chanted for myself. I did know how to chant, and to teach her I didn't need a book, or a CD, or the help of others; I could draw from what I had already assimilated from my own teachers. Instead of driving off to spend my afternoon at the ashram, I was instead nourished by the opportunity to give to this woman in need.

We didn't get off to a good start. She found it hard to concentrate. I waited, giving her patience and focused attention. She began to shed her distracted chatter as we blessed one another simultaneously, looking into each other's eyes and reflecting the sentiments of the words with hand gestures. "How will I remember all of this?" she worried. Desperate to be sure she would remember the words, she reached in her backpack and pulled out a watercolor brush and paper. Sitting on a rock warmed by the sun, she began to paint the words as I repeated them slowly.

December 23 arrived all too soon, when the winter days were at their shortest. My day would be very long. It was early enough in the morning that it was not yet daylight when I arrived at City of Hope for breast cancer surgery. Nevertheless, even in the darkness the beautifully landscaped grounds were discernable as a welcome mat that soothed my soul.

I'd read widely from Bernie Siegel, Andrew Weil, Judith Prager, and others, and I knew about the profound positive impact encouraging words and comforting music could have during medical care, including surgery under anesthesia. I believed that every aspect of my surgery, including conversation among the medical team, needed to be only about my well-being in order to ensure a most positive outcome. I wanted to ask that no gossip or personal chatter take place, as was often portrayed on television shows, and I wanted to bring recorded music, to be played during my surgery, that would ease my spirit, boost my immune system, and promote optimum healing. Could I speak up about my wishes? I feared that a conventional medical team might not agree to my requests or would even ridicule them while operating. And how would I ever be able to pick out the perfect music CD? Maybe the answer was this—the music I needed was already a part of me. After all, I knew chants I could sing to myself.

Upon entering the room where I was to be injected with radioactive blue dye as a tracer for my sentinel node biopsy, I experienced the benefits of my personal music treatments and my thoughts regarding the needs of others. The door was covered in gift wrap and ribbon, reflective of the holiday season. Rather than fear possible carcinogenic affects of radioactivity or blue dye, I knew I needed to embrace the medical treatments I had chosen and visualize them doing the best work they were designed to do. With gratitude I told myself that whatever happens in the room behind the gift-wrapped door is a gift, and I repeated it to the nurse inside. When I saw her name was Joy, I felt that as I did my part to create the reality I wanted, I became more open to noticing the beneficial aspects that were already present. Not only her name but her quality of care was a gift.

The last thing I remember before succumbing to anesthesia was silently chanting to myself, "May the blessings of God rest upon you. . . ." The chant was all the more potent as I imagined the woman at the hot springs face-to-face with me. Though I thought I had been giving to her as I taught her the chant, now that her face came back to me as a gift at this crucial moment, I was reminded that actually we are simultaneously both the giver and receiver.

BERNIE'S REFLECTION

Learn to listen to your heart and not your head.

As I read this story I suddenly had a sense of what Paula was sharing. It was not just about her experience with cancer, but about where she was in her life and where she needed to be. She starts off describing the details of the place where she was and being ankle-deep in a pool of water. She talks about how she was searching for peace even as she judged the other woman. I felt she was coming from her head at that point and not her heart.

Then she shares her experience of teaching someone to chant, and why she felt the need herself. As she does this, one can feel her moving from her head to her heart, the place we all need to pay attention to and find. As she makes this shift, she lets go and begins to move toward just the peace she is looking for.

Paula talks about her depleted years when she suffered from a lack of emotional and physical energy, and how helping another person to learn to chant helped her feel restored even more than going to the ashram for the day. She went there originally to find the flow, and that is what we all seek. The way to find it is not mystical. You find your flow when you help the people before you by doing what they need you to do now. We are all here to contribute love to the world, and she found a way of doing it and was transformed by her actions.

We are all alone in the wilderness, as she was, until we connect with others and find meaning in our lives. She talks about the giver and receiver being the same. Yes, we are all experiencing life and need to realize we are the same at both ends of the rifle.

At the end of Paula's story there is a sense of peacefulness in her words. She is no longer coming from her intellect and describing, but coming from her heart about her feelings and experience. There are no details but the simple truth. She talks about the benefits of what is about to be done and her absence of fear. As you go through life, see every door you must pass through as she did, a gift-wrapped door, and when you do, everyone you meet on the other side of the door will be named Joy.

Love Heals

Ruth Vanden Bosch

It seems like only yesterday that I received the telephone call that every woman dreads. . . . We all hear the doctor say, "I will call if something is abnormal with your Pap smear or lab studies." And then we pray that the phone never rings. Mine did.

It was late at night and I was driving home in the middle of a snowstorm from my graduate class at Western Michigan University. The news came quickly—my gynecologist calling to tell me that my recent Pap smear was abnormal. "Could you come in early tomorrow to discuss the results of your tests?" How could it be anything, really? I felt fine, just a little tired from graduate school, my job as an RN, and a new business I'd recently started. Just a little tired, that was it.

The next morning my doctor told me my Pap smear indicated that I had grade IV adenocarcinoma of the endocervix of my uterus. He'd gone to the pathology lab and looked at the slides himself. I'd need a radical hysterectomy and would lose my uterus, ovaries, omentum, and several of the lymph nodes from my pelvis. Before I could even absorb these words, he announced that I'd need a conization of my cervix for staging, and that the surgery was scheduled for the very next day.

Cancer? How could that be? I cried all night and went to surgery the next day in total shock and denial. Three days later I met again with my doctor, and he confirmed the diagnosis. "If you don't have the surgery, you have less than a year to live." Radiation and chemotherapy would be necessary as well. The reality of all of the information was overwhelming—I would have to go through major surgery that would change my life forever. I would never be able to become pregnant and experience the joy of motherhood and, at age thirty-five, I would experience a surgical menopause. What man would want to marry me if I could not have children?

During the next weeks before the surgery, I went through every emotion in a few minutes. One minute I was hopeful and felt that I would beat this and be fine. The next minute I felt angry and asked: "Why did this happen now? My life is perfect and I have so much to live for and so much left to do with my life!" With a new business to run, employees who depended on me to provide employment, and graduate classes that I wanted to complete so I could fulfill my dream of being a psychologist and a counselor, I just didn't have time for a cancer diagnosis!

The hardest part of having a new cancer diagnosis was telling my family, friends, and employees of my diagnosis. I didn't want to hurt them, I wanted to protect them from unpleasant things. One day I suddenly realized that I always took care of everyone and not myself. I never said no when anyone asked me for help. I had spent my life taking care of the world, and my identity was related to how much I could help people. I had become a shadow of myself and I really had no idea of my true self. I owned a business and never expressed my true feelings. I spent my time becoming successful by pleasing customers and clients and keeping my employees happy. I never put my needs first. I was always tired and never rested or took a day off.

I remembered a book that was required reading for one of my classes the semester before. What was it called again? *Love, Medicine, and Miracles?* I remember thinking at the time that it would have been a help to my Aunt Trudy, who had died of liver cancer the year before. It would have helped her so much. Perhaps it would also help me. Finding the book on my shelf, I began to read it again, this time with a yellow highlighter pen. I also noticed that the telephone number for ECaP (Exceptional Cancer Patients) was listed in the postscript. I called and ordered Dr. Siegel's meditation tapes and his book *Peace, Love and Healing*. Soon this book also resembled a worn textbook, with scribbles and notes and questions in the margins of the book that I needed to answer and priorities I needed to set about preparing myself for surgery.

The book became my guide and road map to understanding my purpose in life and to discover the way back to health. Dr. Siegel discussed the relationship between withheld emotions and the development of cancer. People who smile and don't acknowledge their true feelings and say, "I'm fine" when they are not are more likely to develop cancer and die from the disease. I saw myself in almost the entire book and I was stunned! Being a "people pleaser" and always denying my own needs was killing me!

I listened to the meditation tapes and visualized that I was shutting off the blood supply to the cancer. I also visualized that my cancer was made of Godiva chocolate, and little smiley faces were gobbling up the chocolate as quickly as possible and I wouldn't need the surgery or the tumor would be smaller and easier to remove.

My surgery was already scheduled when my surgeon called to say he had been called out of town. Rather than wait and reschedule, I asked if instead I could have my surgeon friend Dean perform my surgery. Yes, that would be possible! I said a prayer of thanksgiving. Someone who cared for me would be doing the surgery. For the first time since my diagnosis, I relaxed a little.

The night before the surgery, Dean took me out for dinner to make sure I was okay. We went to a fabulous Italian restaurant and ate a large pizza and drank a bottle of wine. We talked about everything except my surgery for several hours. He finally decided that we needed to get some sleep, as we both had an important date the next day! I went to sleep with a smile on my face and didn't wake up until six o'clock the next morning.

When I got to the hospital, I found several of my friends, my pastor, and my family waiting to sit with me until I went to surgery. We passed the time with hugs, prayers, and funny stories.

So funny, in fact, that when the surgical assistant came to pick me up for surgery, I told him that I was having too much fun to leave my room. Dean peeked around the corner and spoke sternly: "We have a date, and I don't like being stood up for dates!"

The surgery went well and Dean was able to assure me that I had a surgical cure and I would not need radiation or chemotherapy. I was discharged from the hospital three days after surgery and returned to work part-time within three weeks.

Due to the hormonal change and the surgical menopause, I was very emotional, crying easily and worrying that the cancer would return. One thing I knew for certain was that if I didn't stop being a people pleaser and continued with my old lifestyle of caring for the world, I would get sick again. There had to be a way to love the world and help those in need without sacrificing my health!

I prayed that God would help me find the answers to my questions. A few days later I received a flyer in the mail inviting me to attend a holistic psychology conference in a city nearby that featured Dr. Bernie Siegel and many other holistic practitioners. I felt the invitation was an invitation from God, and I quickly registered and attended the conference. I also wanted the chance to meet Bernie Siegel.

The conference was amazing. Many of the speakers were survivors who spoke eloquently about how to live a healthy life after cancer. They'd made major changes—becoming vegetarians and making sure they had daily exercise and giving up smoking or drinking alcohol. They seemed to be at peace and continued to seek their health by attending conferences and remaining educated about health issues. I agreed with their healthy lifestyles. However, I needed to find inner peace and stop worrying about my health and the possibility of the cancer returning to another part of my body.

Bernie Siegel's talks helped me the most. He talked about being able to say no when you don't want to do something. This would be a struggle for me to adopt—I rarely said no to any request and I found it almost impossible to stop pleasing everyone. He helped me to understand that my personality was programmed long ago by my family.

My mom was a beautiful woman, and a perfectionist. My father was a minister and a counselor, and as a "preacher's kid," I had to be the example for the children in his churches. It was a heavy burden for a young person to carry. I can still hear Mom telling me that I had to be the example for the other kids and that "everyone was watching what I did." It was no wonder that I grew up to be a people pleaser, a perfectionist, and a "success junkie." I always strived to be number one in everything and I could not accept failure. Criticism was hell and did not "polish my mirror." It was pure torture, and I still have trouble receiving criticism without tears.

Listening to the speakers that day made me realize that I could be "born again" as a new person and "stop killing myself" by trying to please everyone. It was okay just to be myself and have faults. For the first time in my life I felt loved. I had hope for the future.

My road back to good health was rough; there were many potholes along the way. I learned to love myself and say no. I was able to let go of my tight control of my life and let God guide my life. I started a gratitude journal that helped me to keep a positive attitude about my life. Every day I find five things that I am grateful for and say a prayer of thanksgiving. I open my mind and heart to accept my blessings. I know that God is directing my life and that all is good and I am doing the best I can. I don't have to be perfect. I know that God's spirit is within every person I meet, every situation I face, and every decision I make.

Every night I also say thank you for the rough spots each day, as it is the difficult times that we learn from and remember. I know that God is directing my life and that all is good and I am doing the best I can. I don't have to be perfect.

BERNIE'S REFLECTION

Love benefits the giver and the receiver.

As I was reading Ruth's story, the first thing that struck me was the doctor's ultimatum of surgery or only a year to live. He is deciding what she should do and threatening her as well. If she doesn't follow his advice, she's dead. What medicine needs to do is offer options and empower patients. Do I know people who refused surgery, radiation, and chemotherapy and are alive today? Yes, and I don't think it's easy to do what they did. Faced with this situation, I do not know if I could believe and have the faith that they had. They are my teachers because they show me the ways to healing.

My next thought relates to Ruth immediately jumping into a disastrous future with her thoughts and the "why me?" attitude. Again, physicians and others need to help us to live in the moment and focus on the now. While Ruth worries about the future, she also worries not only about her feelings but also about not hurting her family. She realizes what I would feel as I read those words: what a "good nurse" she is, busy caring for the world while dealing with her cancer.

Ruth says, "I never put my needs first." I wanted to scream when I read that. We are not talking about being selfish; we are talking about you living your authentic life. She became what others wanted her to be and lost herself in the process. Ruth was smart enough to know that you can let your untrue self die and start a new life.

She did this by having a team around her to help her get through the surgery. She turned her cancer into a chocolate treat and gobbled it up. Then she used books to guide her and provide her with a road map. That is what we all need in our lives: to find our path and let the wisdom and experience of others guide us.

I love her final realization: "I don't have to be perfect." So to all of you, learn from Ruth's experience, and don't let your true self die while trying to be perfect for everyone else. For your health, drive everyone crazy, be different, be a character, and never ever grow up because it can be bad for your health.

I know Ruth very well; we have done many workshops together. She has honored me by getting a puppy and naming it Bernie. This confused her neighbors who heard her yelling, "Bernie, stop biting my toes," until they learned about the puppy. I can honestly say she has accomplished her goal and is definitely not perfect. Ruth, if you're not smiling now, the nurse has taken over again.

Wildflowers

Sue Pearson Atkinson

I walk the stone dust path of the labyrinth I created in my back-yard, meditating and feeling the rising joy as I pass the sweet pockets of wildflowers tucked into the rock border that remind me of death. This peaceful walk holds no dread. Dotted with the brilliant color of lupine and poppies, I sowed the seeds of the wild-flowers here to remind me of the lessons I have learned from being close to death several times on my own, and of the passing of my husband's mother.

Although Nicky was my mother-in-law, she was a true mother to me in many ways, as well as my great good-girlfriend and a wise woman I turned to often. When I married her son, I had no idea my relationship with her would be one of the most important of my entire life. Deeply religious, she didn't force her way of think-ing on anyone but accepted people as they were, celebrating their gifts and overlooking their flaws. She had an extraordinary capacity for unconditional love.

She'd married quite young, only seventeen, because her par-ents thought she had attracted an older man who would take good care of her. Six babies soon followed, all sons, all in a row. Nicky's husband, Presley, was a man who craved adventure and invention, everything from brainstorming a potato chip factory in Germany, marketing a casino in Bogotá, or roughing it in a high Sierra cabin on the chance of striking it rich in California gold country. A good man, but not around much during their early years of marriage and babies. Nicky felt like the woman in the nursery rhyme, living in the shoe with so many children that she didn't know what to do. Over a cup of tea in her kitchen, years after all of this was behind her, she told me how she'd once cried for an entire month hoping someone would see her despair and give her a helping hand with all those children. What you got back then when you were depressed was harsh—electroshock therapy.

Nicky learned from her own pain and despair that we are all wounded in some way. She looked to God to provide healing salve, and she was transformed. She judged less, loved more, rose to a challenge when she could, and accepted circumstances beyond her control. Diagnosed late in life with lung cancer, she became serene with her surrender as her time on earth ran out.

My own transformation began in a blink of time. Rather than cumulative wisdom born of a hard journey, my gift of peace was delivered in something like a bolt of lightning. At the time, my life was looking pretty wonderful. I had found a beautiful house in the country, with a lovely view of snow-capped mountains and enough land to keep my horses. My husband and I had endured our share of chaos raising five children and keeping two careers afloat, his as a neurologist treating stroke patients and mine as a journalist producing documentaries for public television. The kids were almost gone and the house in the country seemed like a grand reward for our hard work. But just months after making this dream come true, I was faced with surrendering it in a terrifying medical crisis I never imagined would happen to me. I suffered the deadliest kind of brain event—an aneurysm.

On my way to the emergency room, I sensed God was asking me if I was ready to go . . . ready to die and leave everything behind. I thought, "Can I surrender everything including this dream that was now within my reach?" The answer came instantly: I already had everything I needed. My life had been wonderful, filled with people

I loved and who loved me in return. I was suddenly so completely grateful for the fullness of my life. Thank you, God, for this amazing time I had here on this earth. I would say good-bye to the house in the country with no anger or regret that time had run out.

At the hospital everyone around me was in high gear. This was a crisis. The doctor explained they would be threading platinum wires up into the bulging vessel in my brain, sending them up through an artery in my groin. The platinum wires would pack the aneurysm much like plugging a leak in a tire. He told me he didn't know if the aneurysm would rupture during the procedure. It had begun to leak—a sign that time was running out.

I was completely and utterly at peace. A silent message embraced me. Everything was going to be okay no matter what happened. The outcome was out of my hands. I was awake through the entire two-hour procedure and I have never felt so calm in all of my life. I could die. It would be okay. I could live. That would be okay. With the brilliance of the medical team, I came through the surgery just fine. But God's presence in that life-or-death situation transformed me. Every day after was a gift.

Nicky became my mentor for my deepening spiritual awakening, teaching me the value of silence and the practice of going deep within myself to be closer to God. All of this work prepared me for a new health challenge—four years after surviving a brain aneurysm, I was diagnosed with a rare, genetically linked, primary immune disorder. I would require monthly infusions of donated gamma globulin to stay alive. Weak and tired, no longer able to work, I still looked for the blessings in my life. I had friends and family and my beloved horses. I adjusted to my disability and led a quieter, more contemplative life. Nicky provided wisdom and comfort at every challenging new turn my life took. And then all too soon it was time for me to be there for her.

She was diagnosed with lung cancer and bravely soldiered on through chemotherapy. A year later the cancer had spread to her brain, leaving her but a few months to live. Those last months I spent many precious days with her helping her put her final plan into action: putting finances in order, clarifying bequests to children and grandchildren, closing up the home she and Presley shared and moving with him into an assisted living center. I cooked for them both—big pots of chili and trays of chicken pot pies, dishes that would remind them they were loved. Never one for sweets, Nicky even politely took a bite of pecan pie I'd baked while we sat and reminisced about the past and laughed about coping with the men in our lives.

She'd always loved Texas wildflowers, a signature of her home state. It was spring, and her chance to see them one last time. We put her in a wheelchair and helped her into the car, then drove out to the beautiful Wildflower Seed Farm not far away. We wheeled her down the paths, along fields of glorious wildflowers, an incredible display. There they all were in all their glory—row after row of brilliant red corn poppies, a never-ending field of bluebonnets, lupine, purple coneflower, orange poppies, and more.

Those last few months she lived in a state of near constant joy. People from near and far came to visit and tell her how much she meant to them. It was as though all those hundreds of people had lined up outside her door to pay homage to a mighty ruler. Love brought them—she'd become a beacon for so many. Now, as we tucked her in for a nap after our wildflower excursion, Nicky looked up at me and said, "This is the most wonderful time of my whole life. Sue, how has this happened—I mean the stream of people who have come over or called or sent cards, wrapping me in their love and concern—even people I didn't know well."

I glanced out her window at the wildflowers in a nearby field before I answered her. "Nicky, I think it's like the wildflowers— every single flower is special, but the wildflowers multiply and the grand display takes our breath away with the sheer expanse of the beauty. You have scattered the seeds of love over a wide landscape. And now you are reaping the glorious harvest—those seeds have grown in expected and unexpected places, blossoming into vast fields of love."

Nicky asked, "Am I special?" And I said, "No."

"You really know how to take the wind out my sails, Sue."

"I just mean you are no more or less special than any of us on God's earth. We each have unique gifts and free will to make decisions on this earth journey."

I miss her so much. Her legacy of wildflowers grows not only in my backyard, but also in my heart. I thought I had faced my share of serious health challenges, but there is yet a third door through which God beckons now. I fought it for a moment when my doctor delivered the news after a routine mammogram: "You have breast cancer—lobular carcinoma in situ." I thought, "Come on, God, isn't this a little heavy-handed? First a brain aneurysm, then a disabling immune disorder, and now this!" But as these thoughts rolled out, other thoughts rolled in: "The brain aneurysm could have killed me. The immune problem was on its way to doing me in until I got a diagnosis and started treatments. With each of these challenges, I had looked for blessings and found them. So why not now?!"

A year and a half after my diagnosis, things seem to be under control. Mostly, though, I've worked on surrendering. None of us knows exactly how much time we have left. Death has tapped me on the shoulder enough times now that I can say, "Bug off! I'm living every moment without worrying about *you*." I want to live reveling in the beauty of this earth and in the preciousness of my fellow travelers. I want to follow in Nicky's footsteps, sowing wildflower seeds along the path and hoping those tiny bits of life take hold in fertile soil. I don't know if my field of unconditional love will be as brilliant as hers, but I am happy—no, make that joyful—to have the chance to touch a few precious souls. Every time I walk the labyrinth path in my backyard, I delight in the small blossoms I helped create here, each one a reminder that love and joy are not things we use up, but qualities that spread and multiply when we have the courage to let go of fear.

BERNIE'S REFLECTION

What you plant in your garden shows up in every
season of your life.

This story contains a multitude of messages about love for our heart and soul. Sue found affirming messages in the natural beauty of the wildflowers that connected her to her mother-in-law. Nicky found the message of love in religion and passed that message on to Sue. Both of them lived the message to heal their life. They did not feel guilty and think that God was punishing them with their disease. Remember that disease is a loss of health, and allow God to help you find it when it is lost.

We all need to realize the benefits of having more love in our life. Letting love in can accomplish amazing things. When Nicky was depressed, instead of hiding for months, she could have sought nourishment. I suggest you use your negative feelings as a challenge to prompt you to seek the change that will help to resolve your unhappiness and depression. Reach out and make changes and see how your life changes. Remember that there are always solutions if you reach out rather than withdraw into yourself and hide your feelings. When you bond with another person, it helps you to heal as well.

When we nurture each other, we find more peace. Our life is more meaningful and we leave seeds of love along our paths. It is the quality of life, not the number of years, that counts. Only love is immortal. At times, Sue expresses anger and disbelief that she had to surrender her dreams to deal with her health concerns. However, through love, Sue found the strength she needed. She also became aware of the gift of each new day. Most important, she was able to return that love to Nicky in her time of need and help her live her last few months in a state of near constant joy. Nicky was blessed to have such wonderful people shower her with an outpouring of love in her final days.

Sometimes it is our tears that make things grow and blossom. I recall the story of the man who brought water home to his family from a distant well every morning. One container was cracked and so water leaked out as he walked. This upset him greatly and he shared this with his wife. She then turned him around and showed him the path he walked each day. On the side where the water leaked out were beautiful flowers, and on the other side bare ground.

We never know how healing nature can be. A story of a Vietnamese man who had been in a prison camp demonstrates this in an amazing way. He had cancer, and the chemotherapy

and its effects reminded him of his wartime experience, so
he refused the treatment and said he preferred to die. It was
springtime, and he told the hospice worker that during this time
of the year in his country, they went outside and sat downwind of
the flowers. The worker arranged to take him to local nurseries
to smell the flowers. The people at the nurseries showed him so
much compassion and love.

On his return visit to the doctor months later, there was no
sign of his cancer. He said it couldn't survive all the love he had
received. I have written in my earlier books about my landscaper
friend John Florio, who also refused treatment for his cancer,
which I couldn't cure with surgery. He wanted to "go home and
make the world beautiful. So when I die I'll leave a beautiful
world." John died at age ninety-four with no sign of cancer. He did
develop a hernia "from lifting boulders in my landscape business,"
which I repaired. So remember, we are all gardeners. Just choose
your soil and your manner of planting the seeds of love.

Once Sue accepted her mortality, she came to understand
how precious each day is, and now she is truly living her life.
Nicky also accepted her mortality, and made sure everything was
in order before her passing. This can ease the stress on loved
ones, who have more emotional matters to see to. So again
I ask you to accept your mortality and live. Surrender to life and
find your blessings. Surrendering is not about giving up, but
about acceptance and the peace that comes with it. When you
surrender, you no longer fight to maintain control, and when
you love, you will be free of fear. So learn from Sue—get out into
the garden of life and create your Eden.

To Be Alive Is a Gift

Susan Orr

August 2001. I stood in my studio finishing a painting for a November show that would coincide with my sixtieth birthday. Although deep in concentration, I allowed the phone's sudden ringing to interrupt my process. I was awaiting a call from my doctor's office with the results from a recent biopsy on a lump found in my right breast. This was the fifth I'd had in fifteen years. It had become so routine, I was unprepared for the nurse's words: "Your biopsy was positive." In the months following that phone call, from biopsy to mastectomy, through chemotherapy and radiation, I found that both my fears and my certainties were mutable, they did not have to run my life. Cancer was just a word, not a story already written with an outcome already determined. I learned that to be alive is enough, is a joyful mystery and a gift, moment by moment.

Mother and grandmother, I was a woman who had dedicated her life to finding healing and creative solutions to problems in my personal life and in the world. I was an art therapist, an artist, and—true to my generation—from very early on, an activist. In my passionate high school years in the late 1950s, I joined the Committee for a SANE nuclear policy. In 1970, at age twenty-nine, I had my first experience with cancer. My thyroid, a gland that is especially sensitive to radiation exposure, was removed entirely. I blamed it on shadow radiation from Hiroshima and Nagasaki. The doctors felt it was due to the annual X rays through a fluoroscope I'd had as a child, the ultraviolet radiation treatment for acne I'd had as a teenager, and the many barium enemas I'd undergone to identify an appendix problem when I was in college. Fifteen years after these tests, in 1974, I spearheaded Nevada's campaign against becoming the nation's nuclear waste dump. Now, decades later, I had cancer again, and an invitation to do all I could to heal myself, which just might include dancing with "the enemy," nuclear radiation.

There was no escaping seeing my cancer in relation to what was happening in the world. But how would I hold it? Would I look outside to blame again? Like so many on September 11, 2001, I was awakened by the clock radio as it repeatedly reported the horrific news of the attack on the World Trade Center. I dressed to the news of the two other attacks and the Twin Towers' collapse in a rain of fire, torn body parts, ash, and rubble. I was on my way to the appointment with my surgeon to set a date for a lumpectomy on my right breast.

Craving some perspective on what was happening to my one life and to all of us in the world with the deaths of some three thousand at the World Trade Center, the following Saturday I drove two miles to the ocean. A walk on the beach was, for me, a dependable way to find a wider perspective on my life. As I set out, feet in soft sand, the big sky and steady *woosh* of the surf brought some calm. I found a few small feathers. I picked them up, thinking to make myself a healing talisman. A few steps ahead there were a few more. I picked them up, too. As I walked, I came across and gathered over three hundred feathers without ever seeing a bird's carcass. As I got into a rhythm of leaning over and gathering, leaning over and gathering, it seemed that I was in rhythm with the firemen at the Twin Towers sifting through the ashes and shafts of concrete, and that the feathers had fallen from the wings of all the new angels in heaven. My grief for us all was held and nurtured. In a few weeks, as I healed from the surgery and awaited the start of chemotherapy, some artist friends would join me in stringing the feathers for an altar we created to honor all those who had died when the Twin Towers fell.

But first I had the outcome of surgery to face. Would the surgeon be able to do two simple lumpectomies or have to remove the entire breast? I had to surrender to going into the unknown. My daughter sat with me in the pre-operation room. Two years before, in 1999, when she was thirty-nine, she had had a lumpectomy, and has had a recurrence of her cancer since. After my experience with breast cancer, she decided to have genetic testing and found that our family's genes put us at an 85 percent risk for having breast and ovarian cancer. She and I have both now had preventative removal of our ovaries. And she has had a double mastectomy. Sharing this proximity to our separate mortality has given our warm connection an added depth, an undercurrent of understanding.

At the time, sitting by my side, she told me she had been perplexed that I would get cancer at all, being a meditator, eating the way we are all told will prevent the disease, practicing yoga and qigong. Left alone for a few moments when she went to see how much longer the wait would be, I had a transcendent experience, a deep and full knowing that my body was a fragile container, a fragile and expendable container, and that my spirit was boundless and solid and enduring, that I had nothing to fear. Fear did come later, and later again, but I had the memory of this knowing and trusting in the life of my spirit to help me hold any fear that would come, and not succumb to it. Like a locket that hangs over my heart, this knowing is still with me.

Yes, grave concern for me—but in the midst of immeasurable grave concern, I continued to feel for the families, the cities, and the nation, for the consequences of the devastating terrorist attacks. I, like so many, had sat stunned in front of the television, watching the playing and replaying of those images of destruction, shuttling back to my own situation, my own mortality under threat of invading forces, and then back again to the pain and loss of so many. It was a time of mirrors for me. I felt betrayed by my body. I felt anger and fear. All the voices responding to the terrorist attacks were also expressing feelings of betrayal, anger, and fear.

I wanted the country to find a way to respond to those acts of terror, unspeakable as they were, without retaliation. Conflict perpetuates conflict, was my view. If I wanted the country to respond from wisdom instead of fear, then how could I do the same? I took it as a personal challenge to find peaceful ways to respond to the inner terrorists who had attacked my body.

There is a huge old elm tree in my backyard that I think of as a teacher. It has suffered many infestations of pests and has lost several large limbs in heavy winds. Still it endures, standing tall season after season, whispering in the wind and rain, home to squirrels and birds and bugs. As I sat under it one day before chemotherapy treatment began, four leaves fell on the table below, as many leaves as I had tumors. The leaves were all nibbled around the edges. I looked up into the tree but didn't see any others with damaged edges. I did see a flock of little birds chirping and pecking away at small insects. I have a fondness for metaphors and this was a gift of one, showing me how I could see the chemotherapy as the little birds in the elm. It could nourish itself on cancer cells while ridding me of them. For me the chemical cocktail would be medicine, not a toxin. I would invite it in to do its healing work, to coax any remaining cancer cells into early retirement.

Between the surgery and the beginning of treatment with chemotherapy and radiation, I had the art show opening. My habit is to title my paintings so that the titles read sequentially as a poem. The poem that came from these paintings seems to me an anthem of my journey. I called it "A Haiku Quartet." I believe it came from that transcendent moment of knowing that arrived just before I went in to surgery.

Time only visits
Each moment a sacrament
Uninterrupted.

Deep in mystery
Fear can bend light, turn the tide.
Sit still and listen.

Sojourn in shadows.
Rest in uncertainty's fields,
Nothing is random.

Grief, grace and rapture,
All gesture, all resonance.
Love, breathe and believe.

BERNIE'S REFLECTION

We are all works in progress.

Susan's experience connected me with so many significant
aspects of life's experience. She is a painter and I am, too. But
I also feel that we are all artists creating a work of art. Just think
of yourself as a blank canvas, or a lump of clay, and a work in
progress. If your painting or pottery does not look right, it doesn't
mean you failed as an artist. You take your palette, remoisten
your clay, and rework it until it becomes a work of art you can be
proud of. The same is true of your life.

We all need to develop bells of mindfulness. Like temple
bells, the sound gets us to become still, breathe, and find peace.
However, for Susan the phone interrupted her work. What
if when it rang, she listened to it ring, like a temple bell, and
breathed peace for herself and the caller. The bell can be a visual
symbol, too, like a stop sign or a red light. So create your bells
of mindfulness and breathe peace whenever you hear or see
the symbol that connects you to a place of serenity rather than
interruption and agitation. Try it, and you will see as I have how
different your voice is when you pick up the phone, and how your
ability to listen to whatever is said is altered in a peaceful healing
direction.

Susan writes, "To be alive is enough." That sentence has
me saying, "Yes!" Life is a mystery and a gift, but how many
of us truly accept it in that way? We are more likely to say that
life is unfair rather than see that it is a gift. Along with cancer,

Susan discusses the September 11 disaster. How can life be a gift when such horrible things occur? Life can be difficult, but nevertheless, one can still thank God for the opportunity to experience it, contribute, and make a difference. When you are grateful for the opportunity to live, life truly becomes a gift.

So in the midst of the difficulties of life, cancer appeared, and Susan saw this as an invitation to dance with the enemy and heal. She demonstrated survival behavior. Dancing is about rhythm and movement, and we each need to find our pace and step in order to heal. Another example of her survival behavior is her connection with nature. A walk on the beach or to a stream can create a powerful healing environment. The feathers also became symbols for her and became part of a tribute to others who were suffering. The feathers of fallen angels' wings helped her to put her ordeal into perspective. Her elm tree teaches us about survival, too. I have watched trees grow around barbed wire, which teaches me to be able to do that also when something in my life irritates me. Trees know how to survive and their leaves teach us about revealing our uniqueness and beauty in the fall of our lives.

Another symbol is the birds. I have seen this kind of image literally lead to self-healing in other women. The birds can represent your immune system or treatment and nourish themselves by eating the cancer. This type of nonviolent spontaneous symbolism is what I find most effective for people. Again, it should be the person's creation and not my prescription to be most effective.

Susan also was able to transcend her own personal needs and find time to think about how to help the world deal with its cancer, be it radiation, pollution, or terrorism. That is when true healing occurs. When you give love, you heal yourself and the recipients of your love. With love and laughter, you will prevent fear from controlling your life and thoughts. You will find the ability and strength to handle whatever you encounter with support and the inner strength I know we all have.

That Susan's daughter was perplexed about her mom getting cancer when she did everything right was a statement that had me smiling. Remember, cancer can affect anyone. Having a healthy lifestyle can help prevent cancer, but there are no guarantees. Also, as I have said, genetics are important, but they do not make decisions. They are activated by your body chemistry, and that is why I ask people what has occurred in their lives when they develop an illness. This is not about blame but about contributing factors.

In closing, let me disagree with Susan. She felt betrayed by her body, but I can tell you that your body loves you. It works hard to mend the damage that we do. It heals itself after surgery, chemotherapy, and radiation. I have always said a Band-Aid is a symbol that reveals that our body loves us. Cut your finger and cover the cut with a Band-Aid, and a week later the cut is healed and you did nothing but hide the wound. So have faith in your body's love for you and return the love so your body receives what I call a "live" message.

Amazing Final Days

Ann Martin Bowler

My brother, Tom, was a passionate person, a learner. He threw himself into everything that he did. My brother's list of achievements was impressive—winemaker, hotelier, businessman, community leader, artist. I believe he achieved what he did not so much because of his ability but because of his passionate approach to life. Tom's passionate nature served him well when he got sick. He studied cancer treatments and found the one that held the most promise. He fervently held hope for a cure.

Although raised in a strict Catholic family, Tom was a spiritual man so involved with living life that he had not spent much time worrying about life beyond this world. He didn't go to church often as an adult, but he led a good life, and was good to the people around him. He felt that if he treated others well, and was kind and honest, he had little to worry about. But when Tom got sick, his focus changed. He passionately began to consider all things spiritual. And he, once again, had amazing results. I'd like to share with you an experience he had when I was with him toward the end, for I believe you will take great comfort from it, too.

It was Thursday of Holy Week, ten days before Tom died. He had come home from the hospital the day before. He honestly was very low, almost silent, sleeping fitfully most of the afternoon. I joined him in his oceanside room, a small and cozy place he had designed himself. Through the large glass windows the view was stunning, and we'd raised the bed so that he could still see the waves. Sitting by him, I asked, "Would you like to pray with me?"

Shaking his head, he answered, "I am." So I prayed silently next to my brother, who dozed and prayed silently.

Later that afternoon my husband, John, and I were standing by his bed when Tom awoke suddenly. He lifted his head from the pillow and stared straight ahead, his eyes bulging, locked on the far wall. I looked at the wall, too, wondering what he saw. It was just a plain wall, adorned with pictures of his children. Was that what he was focusing on? After about thirty seconds, he flopped his head back on the pillow and said, "It was fantastic! Fantastic!"

At that very moment, his wife, Noreen, came in with the phone. It was the family priest, Father Spitzer, calling to share the news that Gonzaga University had given Tom their highest award for all that he had done as an alum. Everyone in the family gathered around his bed to hear the news. It felt good to see Tom so happy! After things had settled down a bit, I asked, "Tom, what was so fantastic? What were you looking at before?" With tears in his eyes, my brother looked at John and me: "I saw heaven, Annie. I saw God!" He put his head back on the pillow, exhausted, and slept soundly for many hours.

When my brother awoke again, he was somehow different. Now, don't misunderstand me, he was still incredibly sick, close to death, honestly. But for the next few days, until Easter Sunday, Tom had amazing moments of energy, leaving his bed for the first time in days. Off and on his pain seemed almost to disappear. He thanked the people who were gathered in his house. He told them that he loved them. He told jokes. He offered each of us bits of advice. He said words that each of us will remember always.

On Good Friday, John and I needed to head home. Tom rushed out to say good-bye to us. Standing there, he hugged me, then slapped my check lightly, and with a twinkle in his eye, he said laughingly, "I'm going to beat you there!"

It took me a moment to realize where he meant he was going, and to know how to respond. Heaven—he was saying he planned to beat me to heaven. But finally I looked him right in the eye, shook his hand, and said, "Well, I'm going to meet you there."

Shaking my hand, he sealed our agreement, saying, "All right then." Ever the honest businessman, I am quite certain Tom has already met his end of the deal.

Tom died just a few days later. I know that the fine care he received in his home surrounded by loved ones is a partial explanation for his energy. But I believe Tom's experience gave him the grace to be able to live his last days in the way that he had lived his life. Confident of what lay ahead, Tom was truly able to be present there with us. Though I will miss my brother always, I will ever be grateful for having been a part of his amazing moments of grace.

BERNIE'S REFLECTION

Even the blind see when they have a near-death
experience.

The easiest way to maintain a sense of peace throughout your ordeal with illness is to have the love and support of family and friends. Death is no longer a failure, and one can die surrounded by loved ones who can accept your choice to leave your body and become perfect again. When you surround yourself with the people you love and share the memories that you have created together over the years, you can die laughing as my father did surrounded by his loving family. With the help of his family and newfound spirituality, Tom remained positive and open to all experiences and sharing them with others. He embraced his mortality in a way that helped Ann cope with the pain of losing her brother's physical body. He gave her the gift of the only thing that is of permanence and immortal, love.

Considering what comes after life can be reassuring to yourself and your loved ones. I feel that death is not the worst outcome. If it were, I think Noah would have argued with God to get a few more creatures on the ark. From my own near-death experience, as a child choking on a toy, to the stories I have heard from others, I believe that though our bodies may die, our consciousness does not, and it is recycled as new life is created. When we have completed our lives, it can be a wonderful experience to die surrounded by loved ones, knowing death is not a failure but the next step in our healing, where we become dreamless and perfect again. Recognizing that you will see each other again, as Ann promised Tom, reminds us that we can always be with the people we love. For Tom's family, the experience of his vision became a gift and helped the family and children to not fear death, but to understand it is a part of life. When we accept our mortality, we truly start to live.

I'd like to share a story of mine that relates to this. Right after my mother died, a mystic friend named Monica called me. She does not live near me and did not know what had happened. She said, "Your folks are together again and very proud of you. And there is someone showing them around who likes chocolate and cigarettes. Do you know who it is?" I said I didn't know who it was and she answered, "Oh, it's Elisabeth Kubler-Ross. She's the one showing your folks around." That's what makes me a believer, because Elisabeth was a dear friend and a very meaningful person in my life, and she loved chocolate and cigarettes. I believe Monica is connecting with the collective consciousness, which is nonlocal and never-ending. I think it is the same consciousness that allows us to communicate nonverbally with animals, too, but that's another story.

PART TWO

Hope

A Joyous Occasion Is a Joyous Occasion

Dina Howard

I've always felt that one of the great perks that came from marrying my husband, Ed, was getting his beautiful sister Kathy as my second sister. In 2006, with the gesture of a simple invitation at an unexpected time in my life, Kathy renewed my faith in myself and reminded me of the power of joy.

Shortly before my fortieth birthday, my husband and I got the wonderful news that Kathy was going to be married. She was also thirty-nine, and truly deserved her heart-of-gold fiancé, Moti. The entire family was elated as preparations for the wedding began.

For me, there was only one problem. I was in the middle of treatment for stage II breast cancer.

While my heart swelled with happiness for Kathy and Moti, I shed tears for myself. The wedding date was set toward the end of my twenty-five rounds of radiation. I had already endured three surgeries (including a double mastectomy), eight rounds of brutal chemotherapy, and an emotional roller coaster I could not have imagined before my battle with cancer began. And besides all of that . . . I was bald!

I really wanted to be unreservedly happy for Kathy and Moti. Everyone else was. My little girl, Maya, then three, was so excited about being the flower girl that it would be tough for her own wedding someday to live up to this fanfare. My son, Noah, then age seven, was looking forward to being the ring bearer even though, contrary to what his little sister Maya thought, he did not get to wear a bear costume. My husband, Ed, was thrilled about the wisdom of Kathy's choice in Moti and eager to be there for her in body and spirit. But it was just a few weeks before the wedding that I realized that Kathy was expecting me to be in the wedding party as well.

I felt physically and emotionally far away from the events surrounding the wedding. I was already overwhelmed by being a full-time mother of small children, a functioning person, and a full-time cancer patient. Yet I wanted to be there for Kathy, Moti, and the rest of the family. Through the exhausted haze that accompanies cancer treatment and its related stress, I began preparing everyone for the wedding. I bought outfits, made complicated travel arrangements, and booked hotels. I shopped for accessories for the bride to wear with her gown and created a binder for the couple to organize all of the details of the day. My children and I collected large river rocks and painted them with fanciful colors to decorate the park for the outdoor ceremony. Friends thought I was nuts to try to attend, much less to be in the wedding, but my oncologist thought it was doable depending on my energy level and with the caveat that I didn't miss too many treatment days. After begging the overbooked radiation technicians, they changed my daily radiation treatment from early evening to early morning the day before the wedding, and I was good to go.

The wedding was on a Saturday. We live in Northern California, and the wedding was in Southern California—about a seven-hour drive away. The plan was to send my family down by car in the beginning of the week. I would do all of my regularly scheduled radiation sessions and then, after an early Friday morning treatment, I would hightail it to the airport for an 11:00 A.M. flight in order to make it for the rehearsal dinner later that afternoon.

By Thursday night, with my family already gone, I was beginning to seriously doubt the wisdom of the plan. I was tired (no, really tired) and burned from the radiation. I also couldn't quite settle on a dress and was completely flummoxed about how to deal with my shiny bald head.

Despite these obstacles, there were many things that made it worth the effort to be present at this wedding, physically and emotionally. Among the many disconcerting possibilities that come along with a serious cancer diagnosis (especially at a young age) is the prospect of not being around for the important events in the life of your family. I wanted to witness this wedding, see my beautiful children in their finery, and share in the joy that brings families closer together. Also, California was experiencing an unprecedented heat wave. It was 112 degrees in Sacramento, where I live, so just getting out of town seemed like a welcome change.

Friday morning was a blur. My gear packed and in the car, I made it to my treatment, applied more ointment to my blistering skin, and headed for the airport. Once I was on the plane, I adjusted my head scarf and heaved a sigh of relief. I had an hour and a half on the plane to read my book and collect my thoughts before jumping into the family fray that awaited me.

I saw Ed standing by baggage claim at the same moment that the temperature of the outside air hit my face. It was 117 degrees! As all of the festivities were to be held outside, my relief at getting out of the Sacramento heat was short-lived. Also, after kissing me hello, my husband informed me that the hotel we had booked was unsuitable and that he had somehow lost my bag of stuff that I had sent down with him in advance, which contained my shoes for the wedding as well as other wedding-related paraphernalia.

Needless to say, slick with sweat but with big smiling faces, we kissed our children, congratulated the happy couple, found a new hotel, retraced Ed's steps (across the city) to find my shoes, and rehearsed for the ceremony. The entire family shared a great meal in the only non-air-conditioned restaurant in Los Angeles's San Fernando Valley, and looked forward to the wedding the next day.

Saturday dawned clear and hot. Ed and I spent the morning buying extra cases of water and spray bottles for the wedding guests to use to try to keep themselves cool.

By afternoon it was clear that the heat was as bad as predicted: 119 degrees. It was the hottest day ever on record for what

Southern Californians call "The Valley." Kathy and Moti are truly "glass half-full" types of people. I wilt in hot weather under normal circumstances, but with the radiation burns and fatigue, I had to make a conscious choice—I could buckle under the pressure, heat, and exhaustion, or I could choose joy. I could choose to rally and to try to dance at my beloved sister's wedding.

I rallied.

In the sweltering heat, I wore a nice dress and covered my head in a scarf. I wore pretty earrings and, over the scarf, a hat embellished with silk flowers. My children as well as the bride and groom looked so exquisite that it brought tears to my eyes. I walked down the aisle on my husband's arm with my head held high, feeling not like a cancer patient but rather like the luckiest person in the world to be right where I was at that very moment.

At the reception that evening I danced. I danced with my tiny, happy daughter, Maya, her Shirley Temple curls bouncing wildly; with my sweet, handsome little boy, Noah, just old enough to begin to feel self-conscious, and of course with Ed, my adoring husband. I even had the energy to dance with Kathy the bride, with my parents and in-laws, and with old friends. Everyone said that I looked beautiful, and you know what? After a little while I actually believed them. Joy does that to you. Gratitude makes you glow more than any radiation-induced sunburn. The choice of happiness had made me far more beautiful than just what I looked like.

I am so thankful that Kathy asked me to be a part of her special day. I am delighted that I did.

When you are mired in a difficult situation, people might not ask you to participate in a festive event. They don't want to impose or worry about obligating you to do something you do not want to do. They might be embarrassed by the baldness or by the idea of someone dealing with the "big C" as part of their big moment. I have to admit that I was scared; frightened of not having the energy to go the distance, and feeling self-conscious about my current state. But a joyous occasion is a joyous occasion no matter what else is going on. Being able to celebrate with your whole heart is a precious gift.

I proved something important to myself that day. I proved that even when the chips are down, I can do all. Because not only did

I attend the wedding, I did everything that was expected of me and then some. I'd like to think that I did it with a grace that was infectious. And all of this was possible because my sister, on the occasion of her wedding, ironically gave me the greatest gift of all: the ability, no matter my circumstances, to always choose joy.

BERNIE'S REFLECTION

You make your own weather by focusing on sunny or cloudy skies.

What occurred to me is that our reflections are about what we see when we bend over still water, get close to ourselves, and see the truth. So pay attention to your reflections and what you are feeling when you reflect upon yourself, your life experience, and your response to it. I think the stories in this book reflect life's difficulties, and how we can all begin again without the need to physically die, but with the need to eliminate the parts of our lives that are killing us so we can truly live.

As to Dina and her words that we are worth the effort: darn right we are. We are all divine children, and no matter what you may have experienced growing up, you are worth the effort and deserve everything life has to offer you. The bald head is a small issue when you realize there is a lot more to you than a bald head. I think what we all need to do is uncover our true selves and our spirituality and emotions and not just uncover our skin. A bald head doesn't change you, and may lead you to hide yourself, unless you get the message it portrays.

As Dina mentions, your troubles get smaller when you are dealing with cancer. The missing shoes become a small problem when you are living with the experience of cancer. You all know the saying, "Don't sweat the small stuff." Well, after cancer it's all small stuff.

The heat would normally have made her wilt, but not when she chose joy. The mind is a powerful thing, and whether it is about your therapy or the heat, you can choose joy and let it into your life without all the side effects others have who battle the heat and their therapy and see it as burning, poisoning, assaulting them, and worse. Hell gets a lot cooler when you walk through it with a joyful attitude.

Joy brings you strength because when you are joyful, you are in a trance state that enhances your body's ability to survive and thrive. Dina also shares how she looked beautiful to others because she radiated joy. I could see and feel this in the office with my patients. When they walked in radiating joy, you knew they were healing and could feel it in the room. It was like an aura the joy created around them. Everyone who saw them knew they were healing.

As Dina says, "The choice of happiness had made me far more beautiful than just what I looked like." Yes, she was learning how to partake physically and spiritually in the dance of life. Our feelings and state of consciousness go beyond our bodies and affect all the people we meet. So choose happiness, and everyone in your life will feel it and relate to it from your family to health professionals. You will become a gift to them all.

I knew the truth of all this, and Dina reaffirmed it for me and she proved something to herself as well. Remember this: you can choose to be joyful and heal because joy and healing are not about what your body is going through, but about what is going through your mind.

A New Autumn

Margaret Shane

It's autumn 2007, and leftover invisible particles of ash, chemicals, and smoke hide in the late afternoon sky. The dark clouds of soot are gone, but the smell lingers, drifting and clinging to my nostrils and eyes. The sudden, monstrous Southern California fires are contained after leaving many people without homes and belongings. The television news plays in the background as I straighten the living room: a stunned woman walks through the rubble of memories and charred valuables. She still has her family and her life, she says, just not her home. I look up at the TV and catch sight of the blackened scene. How will those hillsides look in the coming months and years? Green again by spring? Perhaps they will even flourish in a new way—there are some plants that can't grow until after a fire. Some seeds need the intense heat to crack them open and give them a chance to expand.

Four years ago another huge fire swept through Southern California. Four years ago a raging fire swept through me, too— quiet, swift, and sneaky, advanced ovarian cancer attempted to destroy my foundation.

I sip my warm herbal tea. Clicking off the TV news, I curl up on my couch with a blanket, feeling safe and relaxed in this moment. My hand touches the soft wavy hair on my head. I'm glad to have it back again. My figure is slowly revealing itself. My face, although still youthful, has a few more lines etched around my mouth and eyes.

My once idealistic expression is more soulful and serene, yet full of hope and excitement.

I was diagnosed in my forties with ovarian cancer, and after what seemed like countless surgeries and rounds of chemo, I'm in clinical remission. Scary as it was to hear the diagnosis, I believe that the fear and the anticipation of the battle and prognosis were much worse. The mystery of it all. Not knowing which side of the hill the fire would come down this time. At times I was discouraged, sad, and worried. However, I decided early on that it wasn't going to beat me, and the gifts that have come from it have far outweighed my actual illness.

My faith in both God and myself deepened. I felt like a large net was holding me up, orchestrated with angels circling, taking turns to catch my fall, to help me beat back the fire when I felt it circling me. Those angels are my family, friends, fellow cancer survivors, doctors, nurses, and even strangers.

A quiet but commanding voice was the first thing I heard after surgery. "You have to fight this," she said. It was Sharon, one of the doctors from my surgical team. Another doctor was in the room, too. His name was Ben, but I nicknamed him "Hair." He had shiny, golden brown hair with blond streaks and penetrating dark brown eyes. "How are you feeling," he asked. I'm thinking to myself, "Lust." I'm also thinking, "It's too bad I have to meet you under these circumstances." My head was spinning, consumed with visions of him driving in a bright red 1975 Mustang convertible with his hair blowing in the wind. His face tanned and rugged, excited to speed down a country road at eighty miles per hour . . .

My family was there for me, too, and my dad's deep, soothing voice interrupted my escapist thoughts. "Hi, Honey, I'm right here." He and his new wife, Roberta, held my hand as I continued going in and out of sleep. My dad, my rock. He has always been there for me with a voice full of reason, wisdom, and comfort. Something wet was rubbing against my cheek. Coming out of the smoky haze again, I saw my brother, Mike. "What are you doing to me?" I asked, slurring my words. "Trying to keep you cool," he whispered, wiping away my sweat with a cool washcloth.

Home from the hospital, my older sister, Cindy, got to work in the kitchen. From my room I could smell the garlic and tomatoes, and hear the clanging of the pots and pans coming out of the cabinets. Meat loaf, my favorite comfort food. One night, I heard my bedroom door open as she tiptoed in to check on me. I said to her, "I don't think I'll ever go outside and play again. Nothing will ever be the same."

"I know how you feel right now," she answered, "but you will go outside and play again . . . you are going to beat this. I had this dream last night that you were sitting on your couch working on something that excited you. You looked so healthy and beautiful. You turned to me and said that having gone through ovarian cancer was the best thing that ever happened to you. It was so real, just like I'm sitting here with you now."

One morning after my last chemo treatment, I was at the LA airport, on my way to the Midwest for a family bar mitzvah. The jolly middle-aged man who checked my bags carried on about how fortunate he felt to be alive and looking forward to a brand new day as he attached the routing tag to my suitcases. He looked at my driver's license to check my ID. "You're very pretty," he said. I smiled, guessing he was fishing for a bigger tip. "Not bad for a two-time cancer survivor." He looked a bit taken aback for a moment, and then he said, "Lady, there's a reason that you're still here."

Cancer is scary, but not as scary as I thought it would be. In the past, whenever someone challenged me or told me I couldn't do something, my first reaction was to feel hurt, and then I would just work harder. I'm pretty sure that stubbornness and a strong will have helped me over the past four years, and will continue to do so. I used to beat myself up a lot. When I start to do that now, I slow down and nurture myself. I see the world through different eyes. My old resistances to receiving what is possible are gone. I've had to let go of some left-brain thinking, so that I can open up more to trusting my heart and spirit. Not looking at the "shoulds" or "coulds," but what's right and true for me. I've had to learn to honor and value myself like never before. The intense heat from the fire has cracked open the seed of my soul. So many gifts . . . my heart is full of hope, love, and laughter. Fighting this disease has helped me find my passion for living fully again.

And now it is autumn again, my favorite time of year. A time for new beginnings, brisk cool air, school-day memories, new romances, and a cup of hot chocolate with marshmallows.

My solid foundation is right here from the fire that ravaged my body. There are new seeds sitting on top of the burned soil for me to sift through and plant. The sky above me is pink, blue, and orange. I savor its beauty. It takes my breath away!

BERNIE'S REFLECTION

Cancer can reflect our true selves.

Cancer reminds me of water in the way it has the ability to reflect back certain truths to you. Both give a reflection of your true self, not from a distance like a mirror does, but from up close. When you become one with the water's reflection of the truth, you can control the forest fires that happen in all our lives. Just as a team of firefighters must work together to control a blaze, you can create a lifesaving team of your family and caregivers. When everyone works together, there is harmony that creates more of a healing environment.

Just as Margaret did, remember to pay close attention to your dreams. They speak the wisdom of the collective consciousness that knows all. In our dreams we can receive helpful messages. Sometimes we can find inspiration in the dreams of our loved one. Whether it is your own dream or that of someone close to you, dreams are here to help provide guidance. It is not up to others to interpret it or tell you what to do. Only you can determine the meaning and message of each dream as it relates to you.

Margaret speaks of the importance of nurturing and not depleting yourself through the fight against the disease. I get tired of all the battles and wars people wage against cancer. It is like giving power to the fire if all you do is think about how to control it. When she stopped trying to beat her disease and started changing her behavior to one of nurturing herself, good things happened. Your body is aware of how much time you spend fighting versus nurturing yourself. When you nurture your body, mind, and soul, growth and healing occur within you. The adrenaline response to fight is meant to help you run from the fire as fast as possible, but you can't spend your life running from danger and expect to be healthy. Rather than thinking about the dangers of the fire within, try to imagine that the flames are related to your passion for life like a candle burning brightly. Your chance for survival is increased as long as there is an inner candle present. When you let the fire represent your passion and not your perceived dangers or fears, you are truly fighting for your life and not wasting your life force fighting an enemy.

Just as Margaret talks of new seeds, remember that life is about new beginnings. So never stop planting and cultivating your seeds of life, and though cancer may be seen as compost, remember how it helped Margaret to find her passion for living her life fully again.

Riding Uphill

Edwina Ford

It was a scorcher. July weather in Bishop, California, is hot; this year it seemed unbearable. I sat in my air-conditioned Honda a second longer, avoiding the heat just outside the car door. The huge weeping willow stood tall against Mother Nature's oven, as did the coreopsis and white lilies in my park-like front yard. *I could do it, enough procrastination, I needed to move along.* Losing the battle, I opened the door and stuck one leg out to touch the concrete driveway, then moved quickly to gather groceries from the backseat of my Accord. With a bag of groceries in each hand, I pushed through the French doors that opened into my small cottage-style living room. The television roared—men and their sports. Tim's bald head showed tufts of new hair, grayer than I'd remembered. He looked small in his big brown recliner. What would the next five years bring? That question haunted me daily, and I'm sure Tim, too. My eyes cut to the television and a view of a quaint town in France. I'd missed stage one of the Tour de France.

"Who won?" I asked.

"Lance—wa—won," Tim said. His blue-gray eyes were tear-swollen and red, but with the smallest bit of composure, he tried again. "Lance won the first stage of the race. Do you know that Armstrong was told that he would never ride competitively again? His former team dropped him while he was under chemotherapy— now he's the winner of stage one!" Tim's lips curled into a smile.

"I'll bet his new team is jumping for joy right now," I said. Inside I jumped for joy, too, both for Lance Armstrong and for my husband. Tim seemed so full of life that afternoon after a long bout with low-energy days in which he did very little, said very little. For him to be engaged in a televised sports event was a big step forward. This felt good—very good.

"He finished the thirty-five-mile sprint race. That looked grueling. One down and twenty more days to go." Tim's voice cracked and his eyes welled with tears again. He wiped them away. There were few times at which I had seen my husband in tears and at a loss for words.

He followed me into the kitchen, leaned against the tiled counter, and continued to share his newly found bike racing knowledge: "Each rider is timed on an individual basis. The race is thirty miles on the city streets and rural roads, and you pedal as fast as you can."

I nodded. "Are you hungry?" I asked.

"No, thanks."

I handed him an apple anyway.

He dashed to the telephone and called his best buddy. "He won. Are you watching the Tour?"

I crunched into my own crispy apple and again handed him the one he'd left sitting on the counter. He took it absently, focused on his phone call. Maybe he would eat it.

Tim hung up the phone, turned to me, and said, "Maybe I will survive cancer and ride my bike again." He swiped at another runaway tear.

The next morning a low mumbling sound from the living room woke me. I'd had a great night's sleep, but Tim's side of the bed felt cold. Not too unusual; he probably slept in his favorite chair last night, I thought as I padded to the kitchen to start my coffee. Yes, there he sat, in his well-used chair, focused on the television.

"What are you watching?"

"The Tour."

He sat holding a steamy cup of tea. And watch the Tour he did—Tim's new summer routine became getting up to catch the live 5:30 A.M. telecast of the Tour every morning, to watch every moment of the three- to four-hour coverage of bicyclists fighting their way through the hills and valleys of France. Days slipped by. On the morning of July 14, the Tour broadcast for the day had ended. I said, "You've really been following this Lance Armstrong guy closely."

"It's so frustrating," Tim nodded toward the television. "Armstrong's in the top five out of one-hundred-eighty participants, and all the Tour ever gets in the paper, let alone him, are small articles on page three or four of the Sports Section?" He shook his head, blinking against the midmorning desert light coming through the living room window. I sat across from him on my overstuffed floral-print sofa, cradling my coffee while he sipped from his tea cup, still shaking his head with frustration.

He looked up at me suddenly, setting his cup down on the table next to him. "You know what? I'm going to give something a try. I'm going to see if I can change that." Tim left the room and I heard him rummaging through old papers, returning with a scrap of paper with a number jotted down. He cleared his throat, took one last sip of warm tea, and began to dial. What was he up to?

He stood waiting for an answer from the other side, and held up a copy of *USA Today*, peering closely at the tiny print on one story. "Hello? Yes, I'd like to speak to your sports editor, uh"—he looked down at the paper again—"Sal Ruibal." His eyes widened in surprise. "Honey, they're putting me through. I can't believe it," he said, putting the paper down and reaching for my hand. His hand felt damp, and trembled involuntarily as he introduced himself to the sports editor. Breathing deeply to control his nerves, he introduced himself and began to explain why he was calling. "Even though many Americans may not be cycling enthusiasts, many have battled cancer. I would like to see Lance Armstrong's story be told from a human interest, or cancer survivor's perspective. I think that others would, too." Tim put his heart and soul into that call, talking fast to keep the sports editor's attention. I listened while Tim pitched his idea. After hesitating he continued, "I'm a cancer victim. That kind of story would be an inspiration for me and thousands of other cancer patients. It's a remarkable comeback for this talented cyclist." He listened to the editor's response, nodding silently for a moment before thanking him for his time and putting the phone back on the hook. "Wow. He said that he'd do a little research, and then see what he could do."

The next day my thoughts wandered as we left for a long-planned camping trip, bumping along the dirt road leading to our favorite campsite. The shiny red truck and our twenty-foot travel trailer gathered thick dust as we drove deeper into the forest for a four-day wilderness experience.

At last we reached our favorite secluded spot. Tall beautiful pines, some twisted, some joined at their base, rose above us as we surveyed the meadow outside of our trailer door. Tim broke the silence with a loud, impatient sigh. "I guess I'll have to wait until Monday to find out if my phone call made a difference. I hope I can find a Friday paper on Monday." He looked out at the trees a moment longer. "Wait, Tom and Terri are meeting us here tomorrow. Maybe they can pick up a copy on the way here." He grabbed the cell phone from his hip and scrambled up a small peak about two hundred yards away. From camp I heard an echoing, "Yes!"

He headed toward me grinning "Tom will bring me a copy of *USA Today*."

On Friday night about six, the sound of a diesel engine nabbed our attention. Tom and Terri were headed up the road. We waited in anticipation while the white truck and trailer rumbled toward us in a cloud of dust. They moved closer. We saw Tom grinning from ear to ear. He waved a newspaper out of the driver's window as he pulled to a stop in front of our camp. Engine still running, he said, "Here, read this." Tim snatched the paper. On *USA Today*'s front page headline, July 16–18 issue, we read: "He Left Cancer Behind." A large photo of Lance Armstrong appeared with the article, his teeth clenched, as he climbed on his bike through the Alps. Yes! Mr. Ruibal had come out with a great story, one that would inspire cancer patients all over the world. Tim had moist eyes when he read that story, as did I. Then, like a kid on Christmas morning, he jumped with a whoop and holler. "I never thought that I'd even talk to the sports editor when I made that call, but this, I can't believe it."

On Monday morning back at the hair salon, Tim told every one of his clients about the article printed in the paper. I'd become an eavesdropper, listening to his stories. I heard one of his clients say, "Tim, how will you ever top that?"

He replied, "Someday I would like Lance Armstrong to autograph my copy of that paper."

Lance Armstrong went on to win the 1999 tour and six more after that, and with every victory the story of this gritty cancer survivor inspired more and more. How much did Tim's shaky phone call help get the word out about our young American hero?

We'll never know, but Tim likes to think that he made a small difference in promoting the Armstrong story to the next level. As for me, I like to believe my husband made a difference, too.

Often the sun shines through the big picture window of our new home. Picturesque mountains with snow-covered tops paint a sensational view. Retired and living on two and a half acres, we fell relaxed in our new life.

Old habits are hard to break, and we still ride our mountain bikes. The other day while out riding, Tim turned to me and said, "I feel great. I survived cancer."

"Yes, you have," I thought, and pedaled harder to close the gap between us.

BERNIE'S REFLECTION

Coming in first is not the issue; finishing what you start is.

In the beginning of Edwina's story, she is faced with the decision to stay in the cool air-conditioned car or step out into the scorching heat. She uses the phrase "losing the battle" to express the inner conflict of wanting to do something versus needing to do something. Edwina wonders what the next five years will bring. No one knows for sure what the next five years will bring. You have a choice when dealing with the unknown: you can focus on possible disasters or choose to be happy. Optimists live longer, healthier lives even though they may be less in touch with reality than pessimists. When you live one day at a time, you take care of the next five years, as shown in the little poem I wrote below.

Eternity

I am asked to be prepared for eternity
How do I prepare?
Where will I spend it?
Fine questions for philosophers
I don't have that problem
Eternity troubles me not at all
I am having trouble with today
If I can master today
Eternity will take care of itself
Eternity from what I know of it
Can't be as much trouble as today
When eternity comes
I'll take it one day at a time

Edwina's husband, Tim, described himself as "a cancer victim." Well, victims and losers do not have many options or hope for the future. But Tim moved away from being a victim by taking the action to call the paper and ask for the editor. He stopped labeling himself in a negative way, and therefore viewing his future based on those labels. Tim made a difference by speaking up about his experience and pain. He wanted to help others who were going through what he had experienced. He didn't sit and whine about what the paper was ignoring; he took a chance.

When you act out of love, you help yourself to heal and you make your life more meaningful. If the sports editor had gone through cancer himself, he would not have needed a phone call to wake him up. When you communicate with others, they can appreciate and understand what you are experiencing. This will help them to get out of their heads and into their feelings. This is why cancer support groups are so beneficial. Those people in the group are living the experience of having cancer, and can listen to and guide others to a place of peace and understanding of survival behavior.

I believe a big part of the reason Lance Armstrong has survived is that he is an athlete. I do not mean his survival is related to his physical conditioning; it is related to his mental conditioning. He knows what all athletes should know: if you are going to be a winner, you have to visualize success and show up for practice. He has been an active participant who knows how important his attitude is to the outcome when competing with cancer.

When Lance gets on his bike, he knows he can be a winner. That is called faith and hope. When Tim says, "Maybe I will survive and ride my bike again," he has been inspired to hope again.

Let me close with an important survival aspect of life, which Tim demonstrated. Yes, he made a difference. You and I make a difference too, and that is what makes us immortal. When we do something that contributes to others, it is like planting a seed that will continue to produce flowers forever. So our acts of compassion and love go on forever. As a young man with AIDS said, "What is evil is not the disease, but to not respond with compassion to the person with the disease." Tim changed the response of the newspaper and, through it, the world.

You can make a difference with a smile, a kind word, or an act. I used to give out buttons that said, "You Make a Difference" to people whom I saw acting in a kind way toward others. You can do that with words, or you can carry cards with those words printed on them and help people to survive. As Lance says, "*Livestrong.*"

Freedom II

Laura Parisi King

My husband, Ed, and I did not have similar childhoods. From the time he was three, Ed dreamed about sailing, scuba diving, and living on his own boat. My childhood in Brooklyn did not consist of boating or scuba diving. A fun day in the water at my house meant that my parents had connected a small sprinkler to a garden hose in our cement backyard, and let my brother, my two sisters, and me take turns leaping through the water as it sprayed up at us. For variety, some days we'd drape the hose through the basketball hoop attached to our garage and let the water rain down on us from above, rather than squirt up at us from below.

No, our childhoods weren't similar at all. He went sailing. I played stoopball. He went scuba diving. I played box baseball. I was a Brooklyn girl. Water sports were not an important part of my life. So how did I respond when he announced his dream of living aboard a boat and asked me to join him? Needless to say, I was less than thrilled. Why change my landlubber lifestyle to one that was not only unfamiliar, but downright scary?

Months passed as I mulled the decision over. At last, with great trepidation, I decided that I would join Ed on this journey.

A case of temporary insanity? Perhaps. Did I do it for love? For the adventure? The challenge? I guess it was all of the above. Mostly, I decided to follow this path in my life because I knew that if I didn't, I would spend the rest of my life wondering what I had missed. This was a once-in-a-lifetime offer. I would have to be crazy to not even allow myself to give it a try. The worst that could happen was that I would find it to be a miserable lifestyle, chalk it up to experience, and return to my old routine. The best that could happen was that I would find the courage to challenge myself, expand my life experiences, and see and do things that few people have the opportunity to be part of.

Ed bought a thirty-two-foot catamaran sailboat that he named *Freedom II*, after his last boat, *Freedom*. We moved onboard in the summer of 1992. We lived aboard *Freedom II* for five full years, and sailed her 21,000 miles, from her homeport at the Timber Point Marina on Long Island, New York, to the coral reefs of the Florida Keys and the Bahamas.

I didn't fall in love with the lifestyle right away. I don't know when it happened, but somewhere along the journey I traded my anxiety for appreciation, my worry for wonder, and my fear for fun. That isn't to say that I had been transformed into Mrs. Ima Boater. I still had many moments when I couldn't relax for fear of what lay ahead. However, I found that most of the anxieties eased as I became more knowledgeable about the boat, about the water, and about my own abilities.

I became addicted to the excitement and the adventure of being one with nature. I loved watching the reflections on the water in the early mornings before any boats had a chance to ripple the surface. I cherished the peaceful calm at the end of a day's run. We swam with dolphins, we petted manatees. We fell asleep to the distinct sounds of whippoorwills, wild boar, and alligators splashing their tails near the edge of the shore.

As with many things in life, along with the good times came some bad times. Our journey included battling terrifying storms, having boats (including our own) dragging anchor in the wee hours of the morning, and having our boat (our home) stolen. Drunks crashed into our boat at two o'clock one morning, and we had a four-foot snake climb onto our boat in the middle of the night. These "bad" experiences proved to be the very things that challenged us and helped us to grow as sailors, and as people.

Every day aboard *Freedom II* was a total immersion into the real world with circumstances that Ed and I had no control over, yet had to deal with. When a crisis occurred, there was no time to ask ourselves, "Can we do this?" or "Can we handle this?" We simply did what needed to be done, and in doing so we learned what we were made of. Cruising under sail gave me confidence in myself. It taught me that I can handle life's challenges.

Little did I know that the lessons that I learned while living and cruising aboard *Freedom II* were invaluable in preparing me for what was to come—my battle against cancer. Sailing taught me to slow down. Before adjusting to life onboard ship, I lived in a world of fast food, one-hour photos, microwaves, faxes, speed dialing, and express lanes. I needed to be moving, doing, going. I had no idea where I was going, or what I needed to do, but I was hell-bent on getting there and doing it. Those years of cruising under sail taught me to slow down and enjoy the present moment.

Under sail or power, *Freedom II* would do an average of 6 knots. At this speed I had the pleasure of experiencing the world as it passed me by, or more accurately, as I passed by it, floating so gracefully in its natural environment. How many people in their lifetime will ever have that opportunity? What a shame it would have been to speed right by it.

Life with cancer literally takes the wind out of your sails. It makes you slow down. It is a life of waiting. Waiting for blood tests. Waiting for scans. Waiting for results. Waiting for the effects of the chemo to pass. Waiting to feel good. It's like being under sail in a world full of powerboats. The world races on, and some days you feel like you're not a part of it. I'm not sure how well I would have handled the waiting, had it not been for my five years aboard *Freedom II*. I learned to have patience when dealing with forces that were beyond my control. I learned that I was able to handle more adversity than I ever could have imagined.

Cruising, like cancer, is a life of ups and downs. One day the sun is shining, the wind is a perfect 10 to 15 knots, and the current is pushing your vessel gently down the waterway. The next day it's raining, the wind kicks up to 35 to 40 knots, and the seas are turbulent and confused. Ed and I needed to be willing to adjust our sails, chart a different course, and change our destination. We had to know when it was prudent to seek safe harbor, anchor the boat, and wait for better weather.

Life with cancer is no different. It has good days and bad days. Some days I was filled with energy. I knew that those were the days to get chores done. Those were the days to do the laundry and the grocery shopping, get together with friends, and enjoy feeling good. Other days I needed to anchor myself and wait out the storm. I needed to allow myself time to curl up on the couch, sleep, ask other people for help, and wait to feel better.

The most valuable lesson that cruising taught me about living with cancer is that bad times, like good times, come and go. And although the bad times are frightening, and painful to endure, they are there to help us learn and grow. The most terrifying days aboard *Freedom II* are the ones that I look back on with the most pride, because I know that I had courage, I remained strong, and I survived.

BERNIE'S REFLECTION

Create a crew of people who will help you to sail through life.

Sailing, cancer, and life are all very similar experiences. As Laura says, the bad times come and go and teach us to grow in healthy ways. From her life on the sea, Laura gained courage and confidence in herself and discovered that she can handle all the challenges that she is faced with. She learned to slow down and appreciate every moment. When cancer took the wind out of her sails, she drew on that patience and a slower-paced life to get through the agonizing moments of waiting. Life is a journey, and sometimes you need to rely on yourself and paddle if you are going to survive and reach a safe harbor. Sometimes you can rely on the wind or treatments to get you through rough waters. You also have to lean on the people close to you.

Once, a doctor with cancer gave me a drawing of himself and his wife sailing. He had his hands on the tiller and sail while his wife was sitting apart from him. The lines of the boat were drawn over her body. It was symbolic of her being tied down and not allowed to decide about the boat's direction. Three drooping dark birds, representing their children, and a little porpoise, his spiritual symbol, looking into the darkness were also in the picture. I shared my theory of his drawing with him and he started to change. His next picture showed him and his wife sitting side by side in the boat sharing the journey. The picture was filled with color, as were the three birds with upraised wings, and a now giant porpoise was turned around facing the sun.

The name of the boat strikes me as an important message: we all have the *freedom* to be who we want to be and live the life we want to live. Don't miss out on life's experiences because of fear. Take a chance and try something new, like Laura did. Laura says that bad times, much like good times, will come and go. With cancer, there will be bad days, but look for and embrace the good as well. Although the bad times are frightening, we learn from them and we grow. The journey over the seas of life can be rough at times, but we are the captains of our ships and the masters of our fate. We hold the compass of our lives in our hands and decide where the ship is going.

Phases of the Moon

Helen Sears

Without the arrival of my husband's prostate cancer, I'd be wedging into old age not only alone but stagnant. I'd become polite, functioning, but I'd be a shell of a person unable to offer anything but neighborly conversation. And so would he. Perpetual new moons with vague outlines and shadows for centers.

A month before his physical that revealed a high PSA, I had a premonition he'd soon face something serious. When he asked me to come home after a three-year separation, I didn't hesitate. Some things fell right into place—his body warmth at arm's length under the same sheet, his curly gray chest hair in the shower, his unflagging exuberance when planning an evening's meal, the body's lower-keyed resting state when assessing problems as a couple rather than as a lone figure against life's chaos. Others weren't perfect. My husband remained distant, if polite, our conversations brief phrases between thank-yous and good-nights. But his dark stares and days of silence were gone.

We had loved cosmically during the years before the separation. Now we needed the small meaningless details of daily living—the tossed salad and scrambled eggs of shared existence. And I wondered what form his stubbornness, part of a buoyant strength that had seen him through decades of corporate life but nearly cost us our marriage, would take next.

After his layoff fifteen years earlier, a nasty political contrivance by his corporate higher-ups that had altered the electromagnetic fields around us, I'd tried every tactic I could think of to start the laughter and loving again. I might as well have cast worms to attract a marlin.

His pushing away had had its own arc—at first embarrassed, then overly courteous, then peeved, as if I didn't get it. He appreciated nurse-to-patient support in the immediate aftermath of the layoff, but he had no tolerance for the perky hostess I'd become. I had nothing to offer beyond meals, polished surfaces, and fresh laundry. Twelve years of bouquet fluffing and simmering his favorite sauces had accomplished nothing.

In the process he discovered that my instinct to nurture had no rational boundaries, tied as it was to a desperate need to please and placate from a ravaged childhood. He inadvertently built a toolbox of sharp comments and looks—blades, awls, and rasps that kept my crippling nursing at bay and protected his cave of despair, but also ground our marriage into sawdust. I left.

Whenever we spoke on the phone or in person on one of his business trips to the mainland, I felt either stunned or sad at what remained—a tarnished affection for an old friend who'd changed. Those years I lived in a cheap, snug apartment were simple and safe, but in a way that made it hard to breathe. On Saturday mornings I'd walk to a park to sit in a rose garden and weep.

Two weeks after I returned to our marital home high on a hill, and exhausted from anticipation, I drove to the doctor's office with my husband. It took forty-three minutes for me to become anesthetized by the waiting room's mute colors, languid from recorded crooners backed by violins gliding en masse around corners and hallways like flocks of white egrets over a pond. I wondered how long it usually took a doctor to share results of a biopsy. When my husband emerged at last from the consultation room, he shook hands with the urologist with the attentive forward posture his corporate years had polished. As he handed me papers and a few shiny pamphlets, I turned toward the exit signs picturing the parking lot and tried to clear my head enough to remember where we'd parked.

He remained silent as we drove halfway up Haleakala, the dormant volcano that gave life to the island and continued to define the landscape. Then he hung up his keys in our house in Makawao, poured himself four fingers of scotch, and headed upstairs to his study, a pattern unchanged for years. I reached for a knife and cutting board to start dinner.

It wasn't our way to discuss events while experiencing them. We were incubators. I washed and blotted fish, placed thick pieces in a frying pan. He would tell me what the doctor said while we ate, before he drained his third glass of wine and fell asleep on the couch.

He came back into the kitchen as I fried fish. "Dinner isn't quite ready yet," I said, and focused on slipping wooden spatulas under the opah to turn it so its flesh wouldn't tear.

"He wants to cut. Recommended next Tuesday."

I looked up. His hands hung at his sides, curved in odd angles, as if about to detach, and it occurred to me to wonder how he'd walked down a flight of stairs and stayed in one piece.

I put the spatulas down and dared touch his arm. It felt warm, as if he'd been in the sun. "What's our next step?"

He showed me what the urologist had given him—a sheaf of papers, all decades-old Thermo fax copies made about the same time we got married. I brought them to my nose and sniffed. No lingering purple smells. "And he said what as he gave you these . . . ?"

"'Stats don't change.'" He finger-licked the salad dressing and grinned in a way that lit his face, a light that shot out from under the brim of our sorrow and illuminated the room like morning. "I'm getting on the Internet."

While I peeled a jicama with broad, even strokes, he scrolled through sites and discovered that patients were encouraged to become their own advocates, that so many approaches and ideas about prostate cancer existed, there was no one format possible for all patients. That night I lay awake a long time. We'd see this through together. Cancer, the great unifier.

He asked for several tests, including a nuclear bone scan, which would reveal whether the cancer had metastasized. It hadn't—by a hair's breadth. To celebrate he took me to dinner and ordered a Caesar salad, gave a nod and toasted the waiter who prepared it from scratch at the table. While a red sun spilled itself on the surrounding water, a breeze lifted my hair between bites.

The next day he requested to see an oncologist, a doctor who could distinguish between need-to-cut and not, and offer a broader range of options. That's when we met Dr. Bobby Baker, newly arrived from Sloane-Kettering Cancer Center with an encyclopedic stack of information and a 3-D imaging radiation machine that could target only the prostate and not the surrounding tissue, thereby eliminating most of the side effects.

For several months before beginning radiation treatments, Murv took Lupron, a powerful blocker of all testosterone, which prostate cancer feeds on. The drug shrank the prostate to make it easier to target, but also made Murv a eunuch. As his belly grew from lack of the male hormone, his eyes got dull with ever-blacker circles, and his skin became pasty.

Privately, I wrung my hands, but when with him, kept a cheery presence. I continued to put fresh bouquets on the dining table, but it was the gnarled jacaranda tree in the backyard I admired. It creaked and flailed in the constant wind but managed to look like moving art.

We no longer competed with one another to create distractions from inflicting unintentional pain on each other. We became a cohesive unit facing down a common foe. I spring-cleaned the entire house. Every closet, drawer, and wall felt my wrath for the invisible disease invading my husband. And yet, within weeks, my role devolved into that of spectator.

Murv never stopped working, or drinking, during his thirty-nine treatments, though he became more and more tired. He still rose before dawn, got to the office by six-thirty, and worked until five. From his manner, he might have been on special assignment and forewarned that any change of habit would undermine results.

He sloughed off any hint to adjust his eating habits. In spite of all the literature telling him to eat small meals through the day and as little fiber as possible, he continued skipping breakfast and lunch, then drank before dinners of self-heaped portions of mashed potatoes or rice with whatever else we had. I knew he clung to routine as proof and silent testimony that nothing had changed.

But in the meantime, his sarcasm evaporated—he no longer made fun of me when I cried in movies; instead he accepted tissues. He started noticing small things, pleasant scents, kindnesses. He started saying "thank you."

It became, in fact, a fascination to watch the layers of testosterone influence peel away. I wondered what behaviors and reactions were my husband and how many were body-manufactured chemicals, and what lay under all that nature- and culture-induced machismo. And what parts of him would be left and if I would recognize any of them. I cooked and cleaned, but also took up yoga, rolling out my purple mat with gestures that would have thrown a skipping rock far out on flat water.

Three months later, he retired and then tried to get life insurance, since his employer's group policy no longer covered him. To our surprise, no one would insure him. Salespeople held out medical reports and pointed at numbers: did he realize his dosages of radiation were the highest ever given human beings? They marveled he hadn't been flat on his back the last weeks of treatment.

Only then did he sit down and shudder, reach with extended lips for every sip of coffee. The "moderately aggressive" growth rate the Gleason score indicated had never meant anything concrete, except as ghostly laughter. Twenty years earlier his own father had been told his prostate cancer would languish quietly in the background while something else killed him—he had a fatal heart attack four years later.

There it was—neither the diagnosis nor treatment of cancer provided our alarm clock's clatter—not even the pasty-skinned snapshots of Murv during that period. But trying to get insurance—trying to sustain a vacuous life as if nothing had happened—that worked to wake us up.

Without substantial insurance we couldn't get enough to cover the balance on our mortgage, so we learned to live knowing one of us would lose the house if the other died. In the process we had to let go of a deep attachment to "home" as a specific place and of the dewy emotional nest that had been our early years of marriage.

That wasn't the only washing away. We now questioned everything that had seemed important, even our beloved jazz. Had that, too, been part of our stultifying politeness, or did it have enough depth to be part of the new territory we explored? We were in a whole new landscape in an uncharted sea. No bit of plant or flower we'd previously plucked and taken into our lives survived its original coloring and nuance.

Reacquaintance took time, or rather, it became an ongoing process, since our paths now often go in separate directions with new interests and challenges. At the same time, when we talk, we finish each other's breaths.

And, while we watch each other age—when we have time to notice between our own pursuits, our noisy or quiet (now mostly produce-based, no-alcohol) meals, the touching of each other's hair or arm as sleep settles in—we are grateful for each additional day of shared life. But more, we also know that whatever the aging process will involve—as well as survival after the other one is gone—the transformations experienced because of cancer will keep the discoveries and celebrations going.

In the meantime, we've never smiled and laughed as much. And we dance under every full moon, that slice of night turned silver by unseen fire.

BERNIE'S REFLECTION

Life is like the moon. There are moments of darkness but
also moments of fullness and light.

I wish more people would be grateful for the full moon of life without having to experience cancer. I know that our wounds can help us grow, and disasters can become our teachers.

Helen shares how the diagnosis of cancer helped her and her husband come together and lead to a rediscovery of their ability to love and laugh. There are many books and articles that show that cancer patients with a sense of humor and who laugh have better survival statistics. Our internal message tells us that we love life and must therefore resist disease.

Helen mentions Murv's drinking. I think that addictions are a search for what the child in us never received in a healthy way. So drugs, food, and alcohol are sought as rewards and to ease the pain of our childhood. But by working on this addiction and healing that pain, they were able to heal their relationship as well.

We should remember that relationships can be an ordeal and a struggle. They require the two people involved to create a third entity, the relationship, which is not based on individual needs. I must add that doctors need to understand this as well and develop relationships with their patients so the experience of illness is treated along with the diagnosis. When their doctor talks about statistics not changing, he is not relating to people. Statistics may help us make choices, but each patient is an individual and needs to be treated that way. Doctors need to listen to their patients, and we need to listen to our wounded family members and help them find the right choices to make. Then we become a unit and work together. When Helen uses the word "incubators," that scares me. If we silently incubate our feelings, we may never learn to heal.

What wakes us up is the acceptance of or threat to our mortality. Then we see a new world. As Helen mentions, Murv started to notice small things. Those things are always right there in front of your eyes. So remember to take the time to see the beauty of the world and creation. The full moon becomes an awesome sight, and the flowers and animals are a wonder to behold.

Helen finishes her story with some important words. We need to understand that life is about never-ending transformation, and never-ending beginnings. She says, "And we dance under every full moon, that slice of night turned silver by unseen fire." Strive to be the sunshine during the day and the full moon at night for yourself and your loved ones.

Opening Up to Life

Kathie Deviny

Today's antinausea meds really do work and I have a healthy-as-a-horse constitution, so most days after my treatment for breast cancer, I had enough energy to work part-time, scratch in the garden, and embark on what I was calling my "new life." I was planning to leave behind the stress and strain, toil and struggle that my tumor had fed on, and embrace the things that it hated—creativity, movement, sunshine, joy, and peace. I was busy concocting the spiritual equivalent of a chemo cocktail.

After I was diagnosed, I felt that my body had betrayed me. At night, my dreams were full of bombs, explosions, and minefields. I imagined that my tumor had erupted out of my chest and that the lava had flowed into my lymph nodes, where it had erupted again. Who knew where it was heading next? Step one in my new life was to negotiate peace with my body.

Once I'd settled into the chemo routine and had come to terms with being hairless, I decided to add to my new life a yoga class I'd learned about. A Seattle organization called Cancer Lifeline offers it free to anyone who's been bit by the cancer bug, no matter if they're still in treatment or finished years ago. Seattle Yoga Arts, which hosts the class, was near my home, and I was nervous as I neared their doorway. There were people I didn't know there, who probably already knew each other. Sure, I'd exercised before, but what I'd be doing was 180 degrees from my familiar but temporarily impossible step aerobics.

And I had tried yoga before. A four-session yoga class twenty-five years earlier had left me with memories of being upside down a lot and consequently dizzy a lot, of trying and failing to touch my toes and assume the lotus position. Now I was fifty-one with a bad case of chemo fatigue, a right arm and shoulder that didn't work very well, a tender surgical site, and creaky body parts.

I was warmly welcomed, and of course wasn't the only newcomer. There were about ten of us, ranging in age from early thirties to late sixties, in various stages of treatment, recovery, and hair status, standing awkwardly in our loosest workout clothing. Our teacher, Lisa Holtby, had founded the first all-volunteer yoga benefit event that had gone on to raise $400,000 nationally for breast cancer research. Cancer Lifeline invited her to develop and teach a gentle yoga program for their clients. The gratitude I felt dispelled my remaining nervousness.

We began and ended the class lying on our backs, supported by mats, blankets, and bolsters, relaxing and breathing. Lisa used the Sanskrit word *savasana* to describe it.

I called it pure heaven. I used to think that slumping into a recliner or sleeping on an expensive mattress provided all the support I needed. *Savasana* taught me that my body loves to relax into the firmness of the floor or mat. When we lie on our backs with our hands facing up, we're open to the universe. I wonder if that is the real reason that sunbathing is so popular. It's one of the few socially acceptable ways to achieve this openness.

After *savasana*, we sat in various stages of cross-legged-ness and opened up even further, about how we were feeling, how our treatments were affecting us physically and emotionally, and which parts of our bodies needed stretching, strengthening, relaxing, or being let alone. This was also the time to announce an all-clear CT scan, the emergence of yet another side effect, the need for more surgery, the appearance of a new tumor. What a relief to be able to unburden to sympathetic souls, and what a privilege to be able to support them in turn.

After that, Lisa taught us a variety of poses, called *asanas* by those in the know, showing us how to adapt them to our own level of stamina and strength. Some of us had off-limits areas—legs and arms swollen by lymphodema; chests, abdomens, and necks tender from surgery. Some of the poses we sat out. Others became possible through creative use of chairs (the better to twist and bend in), blocks (easier to reach than our toes), bolsters (great to ride), and belts (too many uses to list).

The poses that involved "chest opening" were my favorites. In this safe environment, I was able to lie on my back, supported by a bolster, with my resculpted chest higher than the rest of me. Or standing, I practiced bringing my shoulders back, hands clasped behind me, and "leading" with my chest, the reverse of my lifelong hunched-shouldered posture.

During sharing time, I asked Lisa when we were going to learn how to do the lotus pose. She gazed at me. Then she said some words that translated to, "Kathie, that's a long way down the path." I didn't feel chastened, because I was learning about "beginner's mind," which gets to ask anything it wants. As I contemplated the words "path," and "long way," I recognized her unspoken promise, "but they're waiting." Yoga practice, which I had imagined as a jump start to my new life, would involve sticking around for a while.

Long after my official treatment was over, many poses remained beyond me: squatting, anything that resembled a triangle, and most things we did on our knees. Mine jumped around like hot potatoes, they were so tender—which I suspected was a lingering effect of chemotherapy. My oncologist said probably not, so I asked the class what they thought. Lisa offered to consult the medical advisors for Cancer Lifeline. Turns out I had asked in the right place—the word came back that touchy joints were often a side effect. That made it easier for me to be patient, and sure enough, six months after treatment was over, only twinges remained.

Each of us was skilled in a different way, and had poses that came easily. My legs hadn't lost their strength, and loved bridge pose (on my back, feet on the floor, and butt in the air). I was also proud of my ability to navigate my "core body" up and down on the mat, the yoga version of ab crunches. No matter what poses we'd struck that day, after a session with Lisa, we yoginis glided from the studio like queens.

Another favorite was mountain pose, or *tadasana*, which is what your mom *really* meant when she told you to stand up straight. I became increasingly comfortable using the Sanskrit terms, saying "*asana*" instead of "pose," or "*pranayama*" for breathing practices. Needless to say, we all preferred "*savasana*" to "corpse pose."

One of yoga's rituals that I grew to love was giving the Sanskrit greeting, "*Namaste.*" Every so often, mostly in movies, I'd seen people place their hands together over their heart and bow to another person, but had never stopped to think what it meant—that the divine in me honors the divine in you. Without fail at the end of each class, seated, we bowed to each other, said, "*Namaste,*" then some of us bowed all the way to the floor, or as near as we could get, arms outstretched, palms together, full of gratitude. Some of us sat it out, or substituted our own gestures.

Nine months after I started, Lisa announced that she would no longer be teaching the class. How could anyone replace our Lisa? She couldn't, but Denise, our new teacher, could and did transform our practice, not to a better place, but to the next place. Grounded in Lisa's strength, wry sense of humor, and conviction that our limitations did not confine us, we were ready to receive another woman's warmth, emotionality, and dedication to serving us.

With our new teacher, the first thing we noticed was that our sharing time lengthened and deepened. A few of us fretted that we'd be denied our elixir of relaxation, breathing practice, stretching, and strength poses. Besides, I'd mostly confined what we now called "circle sharing" to saying I needed a pose for my aching back or reporting on my latest medical test result. I hadn't felt comfortable opening up about actual emotions. Prompted by Denise's intense interest and desire to learn what we needed, one day I found myself saying, "I'm real sad today; my oncologist is moving to a new practice." "I'm sad too, I miss my sister," said a quiet voice next to me, and everyone understood. The tears became part of our practice.

After minor adjustments, we learned that we could take as much time as we needed to share with the circle, as long as we stopped this side of shooting the breeze. Denise continued our beloved *savasana* periods; we would have gone on strike if she hadn't. She talked to us quietly while we lay back, reminding us to notice our breath, to observe the chatter of our minds, to acknowledge and accept whatever turmoil our bodies or emotions were in. Her words were like tinctures, which we drew upon for physical, mental, and emotional pain relief. We were like children taking naps on our mats while teacher told us a story. It lulled us into deep relaxation, sometimes into sleep if that's what we needed.

Gradually, gradually, I accepted my breath as part of me, a part that wanted to help me heal, a part that could relax me, help me be strong, stay the course with me. Knowing how to take deep, three-part breaths came in handy when I was on the receiving end of blood draws, chemotherapy, and radiation, turning what seemed like invasions into rescue missions. Yoga practice certainly hasn't turned me into a flexible, enlightened goddess. It's done something much better—it's sustained and supported me in the life I've been given.

I've learned that in life, as in yoga practice, when you're sad, tired, or nervous, there's at least one "pose" that's not beyond you. If you can't manage a downward-facing dog or even a smile, your intention and your breath are your sure companions.

I'm now friends with my body—all of it: my guts, my skin, my creaky bones, my left breast, my right breast, its scar, the scar under my armpit, my armpit—you get the idea. Through the poses and the breath I touch them, give them a squeeze, and they talk back—growling, cracking, expanding. If there are any tumors in there, they have to play, too. And one recent day, during *savasana*, as the rest of my body sank into the ground, the place on my chest where the tumor had been twitched twice, then settled down with the rest of me.

BERNIE'S REFLECTION

Act like a survivor.

When you read books about cancer written many decades ago, before more advanced treatments became available, the psychological factors were discussed in greater detail. Statements like cancer is "growth gone wrong" and factors such as being unloved by parents, being childless, and facing retirement all related statistically to the onset of the disease. Now these factors are often overlooked because of the technology available. I think both are important; scientific and emotional elements need to be integrated into the care of the cancer patient.

That's why I agree heartily with Kathie's statement about opening up to life and eliminating the stress and strain that the tumor feeds on. She acts like a survivor when she decides to embrace creativity, joy, and peace—all the things that her cancer hated. I agree with her words and actions because I believe our attitudes and thoughts become our body chemistry.

She mentions feeling that her body betrayed her. The body doesn't make the decisions, we do. Our body is simply responding to the messages our genes receive. The solution and key are simply to do what she decided to do, and that is to embrace life and enjoy the physical benefits that come with the embrace.

Just as she enters a yoga class without fear of not doing it right and being a failure, so it is with embracing life. It is not about judging yourself or being a failure if you are not cured. It is about participating and having a life of your own, a vital choice for many women to make. Her early dreams were full of danger and things to fear. That was her unconscious challenging her to face her mortality and make peace with her body and the dangers that come with it. The more we honor and love our bodies, the longer they will survive. It is our home for this lifetime, so care for it as you would your home when it needs repairs.

In her yoga class she begins to connect with a higher state of consciousness. I think we can all do this, but it is hard and frightening for some people to stop doing things, be silent, be still, and listen. When you stop distracting and numbing yourself, you will hear what lies within you. You will see what you need to face, and you will connect with a wisdom that transcends your usual state of consciousness. To meditate is to know yourself and connect with universal wisdom and consciousness, an incredible resource available to us all.

Participating in a group is empowering, too. It is a room full of natives who can listen to one another and not try to solve everyone's problems. They strive to understand what each is experiencing, and thus help them to find their solutions. Tears are okay; the group's response is to hand you a tissue rather than reassure you that everything will be all right and you don't need to cry.

Kathie understood the message when yoga gave her something to feel good about. Yes, that's what we should all be doing: listening to our hearts. We need to say *namaste* to our inner selves and honor ourselves rather than be critical and filled with guilt, shame, and blame because of our past experiences. Kathie talks about breathing: inhale, inspire, and give yourself life. When you focus on your breathing, you will find your mind clears itself and has no room for fear and uncertainty. You are in the moment and alive, and not expiring but inspiring yourself.

So make your life a yoga position. Find the right pose for yourself to live in and use it to help you rise above all your fears. Having your friends, relatives, and support people around you and your body helps you, and they become part of your team and yoga class—all living and working together for the same purpose: your healing. You can be their instructor and guide and help yourself and your team to achieve harmony.

Lemon Meringue

Padgett Tammen

Cancer. I was thirty-one and pregnant when I got the diagnosis. Old enough to understand the gravity of my doctor's potent words, but young enough still to possess that "it won't happen to me" ideology, which young people quite frequently do. Offered an abortion so that I could begin treatment, I quickly declined. I knew in my heart that with faith, my baby would arrive safely. I didn't fear death, but instead worried that I would never get what I wanted most in this life before it was too late.

So then, I waited. Waited for the baby to be born. Waited to find out what would happen afterward. To the world, I appeared a healthy pregnant woman but secretly, I knew the truth. I was a woman with a dirty secret—holding the cancer diagnosis information in a dark corner of the back of my mind, right next to the memories of loves lost and certain failures.

I thought my wait was up when my beautiful, healthy baby girl entered the world, right on schedule. And I lived, for a few weeks, in a glow of what *could be*. In denial, the cancer diagnosis seeming like a bad dream—and maybe it was?—I woke with a start a few weeks later when the phone rang.

Eight months had passed since the diagnosis, and I plunked my new bundle in her bouncy chair as I soaked up the grim news like a dirty old sponge. "The cancer has gone too far; you need a hysterectomy, if you want to live," my doctor said. My baby daughter, sensing the danger, projectile vomited as I hung up the phone.

Although I am a positive person by nature, the prognosis hit me like a swift gust of wind. We weren't done with our family yet—my husband and I wanted three children altogether. I especially wanted a son. But in a family of girls for several generations, with a hysterectomy looming, it looked like my dream would be quickly swept away. Fatigued from new-baby duties, and with cancer growing inside, I had to let go. Fiercely independent all my life, I knew I couldn't make it on my own anymore. My doctors, my mom, and my husband took over. Although I remember this period as a very dark time, it was lit by the bright people I had all around me. I moved slowly ahead as their light showed the way.

During the moments preceding the surgery to remove my cancer, my surgeon stopped to talk with me, to explain the process I was facing. "Any questions?" he asked.

I nodded slowly. "Yes. We want to have more children," I said, fully expecting him to just say, "I'm sorry," or "You can always adopt." Instead he nodded back at me. My heart lifted at his next words.

"Although I'll remove your uterus, I'll preserve your ovaries and keep them safe—in the future, you can do in vitro fertilization with your eggs and your husband's sperm, and create embryos. You will need a place for the babies to grow: you will have to get a surrogate mother. But it is possible for you to have more children. It's possible."

"It's possible," I said to myself as my eyes closed in the operating room. It is possible. What a remarkable gift I'd just been given. I've sometimes wondered if perhaps this gift of hope was greater and more powerful than the procedure he performed on me that day.

I'd never really feared death, but in the dark recesses of my thoughts, I realized that my cancer might come back at some point. Now as a mother, I considered what death would mean. In my imagination I saw my husband and daughter traveling through life the best they could without me. I saw them alone at a park, my husband gently pushing my daughter on a swing. With that vision, I realized that another family member, a sibling for my daughter, would change the family dynamic and improve their chances for happiness. Now I saw my husband, my daughter, and another child, living as a family of three, sharing and caring. Not replacing me, but living as a more solid unit.

As I selfishly wanted another child for me, especially a son, something inside me wanted another family member for them even more. Then I realized that something was love. And this love gave me purpose.

"Life gave me lemons," I thought. "I will make lemon pie!"

Two years later we jumped for joy at the news that our surrogate was pregnant. And as my dream of a son showed up as a reality at our twenty-week ultrasound, I glanced at our surrogate's face for a minute when I turned my eyes from the ultrasound screen. Flat on her back, with my future inside her, she smiled. And at that moment, I realized that it was her breezy, giving spirit that blew the clouds from my darkness. Not only was I receiving the gift of a son, I was getting a wonderful friend at the same time. Her love rained down on me and I soaked it up like a parched desert flower.

It's hard for me to describe in words what I felt the moment my son entered our world, from his cozy safe spot inside the generous woman who cared for him during his nine-month gestation. For here I was at the hospital again, surrounded by medical people and bright lights, like I had been for my cancer surgery just three years before. But this time, my surrogate was the one on the bed-table, and as I stood nearby, the bright yellow sun shone down on me through the labor-room window.

As he cried his first cry, I moved forward to cut the cord, like a father might do under regular circumstances. The silver medical snips wiggled, my hands were shaking. And as I held my new child, I realized that yes, cancer had changed my life. But with faith, bright shiny people to help me, amazing doctors, and a woman willing to help create a new life with my husband and me, still, I could prepare my lemon pie. It may ordinarily take *two to tango*, but to build my family, it took a team of many, including: my husband, myself, our surrogate, and God. For you can plant a seed, but you can't make it grow.

Yes, we created our pie: my precious new son. I also got a surprise: the love and friendship of my surrogate. Some people get an unexpected gift and call it the "icing on top of the cake." But for us, our experience with surrogacy after cancer was a thick layer of meringue on top of our lemon pie. How delicious!

BERNIE'S REFLECTION

When life hands you lemons, make a lemon meringue pie.

There are many people who do not fear death, but instead fear that they will never really live and accomplish their dreams. When faced with cancer during her pregnancy, Padgett did not allow her disease to stop her from being what she wanted to be: a mother. Even though cancer took away her ability to physically give birth, it did not take away her chances of having more children through a surrogate mother. Her desire to be a mother led her to a meaningful and lasting friendship as well.

Survivors ask for what they need when they need it. They are not hiding their feelings and needs to please everyone else. They seek answers. Padgett questioned the doctor in order to ease her fears and learned that she could have her ovaries preserved, which would allow her the possibility of more children. She also shares that her loved ones became the light that lit her way. They responded to her needs out of love. My hope is that you will educate your family so they all do things for one another out of love and not guilt.

You can see how she kept her power and found that wonderful, empowering survival quality, hope. I was criticized years ago for giving false hope. But there is no false hope. Hope is real and is needed for survival. False expectations and beliefs can exist, but hope is real. It takes a survivor personality to be willing to step forward and to know that dying doesn't make you a failure, but never living your life can. Life is about endings and new beginnings and turning lemons into lemon pie. Look for the little miracles in your life that will be the meringue.

The Touch

Ann Stephens

Everyone knows they are going to die; cancer patients believe it. How do people go on living when they know they are going to die?

I was in the office of Dr. Back, an oncologist—crying. Everything had happened so quickly. It had been just two months earlier, as part of a routine medical checkup for people over fifty, that I had undergone a colonoscopy, a procedure where the entire colon is examined with the aid of a small camera. The result: cancer! I had surgery to remove the cancer and part of the colon. I was now in the doctor's office to consult about chemotherapy. The options and impact of the upcoming regime as he described it were overwhelming. The tears welled up before I could stop them.

Dr. Back had probably seen these tears before. He seemed to know that healing was more than physical. He got up from his desk chair, knelt down in front of me, and took my hands while I continued to cry. His simple touch me gave me a feeling of relief and comfort.

My thoughts went to an incident twenty-five years earlier, when I, too, held the hand of a cancer patient—my mother. I'd always thought that if I got cancer, it would be breast cancer like hers. I'd long carried this image of cancer making one not physically whole. Back then, the biopsy and surgery to remove the breast, if needed, were done at the same time. When given her diagnosis, my mother immediately expressed her concern not over the reality of having cancer, but over losing her breast.

I was with her when she had the surgery. She'd been given a sedative, and in the final moments before she was being rolled into the operating room, she reached over and took my hand.

"Ann, what I want most of all is for you to have someone. Someone you care about. Someone who cares about you." I smiled down at her, touched by her words. She was worried because I was engaged, and had been for a while, without plans to marry. I squeezed her hand in answer, not letting go until she was being taken into the surgical room.

While she was in surgery, I sat alone in the waiting room, praying and making the "deal." If my mother would come from surgery cancer free, then I would get married. "Please God," I kept chanting. "I promise I will marry if you let me keep my mother."

Hours passed. Finally the doctor came out. "She's recovering nicely from the surgery. The biopsy indicates the growth in the breast was benign. It was not cancerous, but some of the lymph nodes were. We removed them and she should be fine. We will need to monitor her on a regular basis." Had God heard my prayer then?

As the months and then years after that surgery followed one after the other, the doctor's prognosis was accurate. My mother never had other signs of cancer. I kept my part of the bargain with God—I did get married, soon after her surgery. I loved my husband, but the deal I'd made about getting married was always somewhere in the back of my mind. I didn't want to tempt God to take back my mother's health.

The thoughts of my mother faded and I was back in the present, weeping in Dr. Back's office. I looked up from my tears and saw my husband's face. I knew that look well. Worried and caring about me, as I had been for my mother. He'd come to the consultation with me that day so I would have a second set of ears to hear what was being said. I did not have breast cancer, but colon cancer. The feeling of not being whole, however, was still there. I had always been the strong one. Now I was the one who needed to be touched, to be reassured.

"Why was this happening to me? Why do I have cancer?" I silently asked God. The reminder of the "deal" prayer I had made many years ago for my mother did not seem right. I was a good person, with a balanced life. What kind of a deal could I offer him this time? I couldn't think of anything I could offer up.

The tears continued. So did my thoughts about God. Without knowing why, I found myself asking Him for the strength and courage to handle whatever would happen. I realized all of a sudden that this was also how my mother had spiritually dealt with her cancer. When she reached out to me that day, expressing not her fears about the operation, but instead her wish for me to marry, she was thinking of someone other than herself. When she focused her physical recovery on the possible loss of a part of her physical self, she was looking to the future where she had survived the cancer. She was being strong. She realized her mortality, but accepted that it was not something she could control. She was putting herself in God's hands.

I looked at Dr. Back. I looked at my husband. My husband's expression reflected gratitude at a doctor who would be supportive of the entire person. Serenity then engulfed me. I realized I was experiencing God at that moment through the kindness, expertise, and understanding of Dr. Back. I would get the strength I would need.

Coming to grips with one's mortality, especially at the same time dealing with physical limitations and the impact of chemotherapy, is difficult. Spirituality includes an examination of the world beyond one's self. With one gentle touch, Dr. Back reminded me of this. He was not someone I had known before, yet he could and did reach out.

Even with six months of chemotherapy and a year beyond that with no sign of colon cancer, I still found myself sometimes returning to those "why me?" feelings. Although I was grateful for the love and support of my family, my friends, and the oncology team, and grateful for my good health, my belief that God had wanted me to have this cancer challenge was still hard to accept.

I was at the receptionist desk, checking in for my regular fol-low-up appointment with Dr. Back. There had been a scheduling mix-up. Another patient had shown up for a last-minute appoint-ment that had not been properly recorded. He responded with the importance of needing to see Dr. Back. He was in the late stages of the cancer and had expected an appointment in hopes of par-ticipating in a field trial.

"I'm not in any hurry," I said. "You can have my appointment time."

The new appointment times got made on the spot and then we sat, talking, in the waiting room. We had an immediate bond of shared experience. The nurse called his name and he stood up. Hesitating by the chair, he reached out and put his hand on mine. "Perhaps the kindness and support we receive when going through a challenge in our lives like cancer, is a way for God to leave us with a good memory of what life is about."

I had been touched again—physically, emotionally, and spiritually. I was where God wanted me to be—not just for this patient, but also for myself. Like all of us, I don't know what the future holds. I might have a relapse or I might stay cancer-free, but that is up to God. That is how a person lives when they know they are going to die.

BERNIE'S REFLECTION

Eventually we will all die, so I suggest you do not waste time trying to avoid death, but choose to live instead.

When Ann talks about the options and impact of therapy being overwhelming, my thought is to tell you to ask your doctor questions and seek advice from people you trust. The unhealthy way of dealing with cancer is to deny your needs and never ask for help. From all of this information, you can then make your own decisions, like a true survivor. If you ask questions, you will get more information from your doctor about why he or she is recommending the treatment. Most patients are submissive and never question the doctor, which is not survival behavior.

Naturally, Ann felt incomplete after receiving her diagnosis. Fortunately she had an understanding doctor who reached out to her with something as simple as a touch, and was able to provide comfort and healing. This minor yet powerful gesture opened the door for Ann's mother and husband to continue to help her throughout the remainder of the healing process. There are no adverse side effects to faith, hope, joy, and love.

It is interesting how many people mention that their parents have had cancer, too. We need to remember that we are not our parents. Being aware of the increased possibility of cancer is important, but cancer is not determined by genetics alone.

Ann's experience in the waiting room shows how she took her doctor's kindness and shared it with someone else in need. When we act with compassion, it is meaningful; when we come from our hearts, it makes an enormous difference to those who are suffering, especially when we show someone that we really care.

Another Kind of Miracle

Jennifer Sander

It was a beautiful, clear spring day when Laura, my best friend for the last ten years, called to say she was dying. "The doctors say it's in my brain now, and it won't take much longer."

Thirty-seven years old, the mother of two young children, and the doctors were right. She died the following November.

"It wasn't supposed to turn out this way!" I shouted at God, shaking my fist in rage. "Laura should have had a miracle. Damn it, she deserved a miracle."

She was first diagnosed with breast cancer at thirty-two, a shockingly young age for such a vicious disease. The younger you are, the more virulent the cancer. When Laura first told me her news, I, being an author, sat down to write an inspirational novel for her.

In my novel she was a character who'd had cancer many years before, a strong and resilient woman who'd beaten the odds and survived. As I finished chapter after chapter, I would call her to read her the story of her survival.

Although I may still finish that novel even though Laura didn't make it, I soon put the novel aside and embarked on a more practical writing plan. Along with Jamie Miller, another friend of Laura's, I began to work on collecting stories of Christmas miracles. Not only would a collection of Christmas miracle tales find an audience, I thought, but it would also bring in some money for Laura and her husband.

Jamie and I interviewed many people who had experienced miracles at Christmastime, and then we wrote up their stories. Laura kept track of the administrative end of the project, and the book we three created, *Christmas Miracles: Magical True Stories of Modern Day Miracles*, became a national best-seller.

How wonderful it was to be able to spread the word about the incredible things that can happen when we open our hearts and believe. Interview after interview reminded me that miracles are everywhere, if you just open your eyes to the mystery and wonder of life.

I had a secret goal during the miracle book project. I believed with all my heart that if Laura was involved in this miracle project, if she lived and breathed the idea of miracles day in and day out, if she helped to spread the word that miracles can and do happen, then she, too, would be given a miracle. The hand of God was everywhere in these tales. I trusted that the same hand would reach down and allow her to stay with her children, to be the mother they needed her to be.

Our one Christmas book turned into a series of five books on miracles. But all the while, as our books grew more popular and we gathered more stories of miracles, Laura grew sicker. Five years after she was first diagnosed, she died. With the final book we did together, *Heavenly Miracles*, she was able to talk to people for the months before she died about heaven, and about how earthly love transcends the bonds of life.

For some time after her death, I was furious with God. Why, after all of the good that she had done in her life, did God allow her to die? Why didn't she get her miracle?

The answer came to me on another clear spring morning, an eerie twin to the day Laura had called with her devastating news the year before. As I looked out my office window at the blooming azaleas and the day lilies hanging heavy from the weight of their flowers, I suddenly realized that there had been a miracle for Laura after all: I hadn't noticed the miracle of the last few years because it wasn't the one I wanted.

I wanted Laura to live. That was what I was asking from God, and anything else was unacceptable. But God knew all along that Laura would die, so God gave her the miracle she would need. She would need help with her children, so he gave her a circle of friends who would pitch in. She and her husband would need help with their finances, so he sent the miracle books project and allowed her to earn an income that would not require her to spend time away from her children in her final years. She would not live long, so he gave her a way to have an impact far greater than most people have in their first three decades. Her name will live on in her books, and even after her death she will continue to inspire others in their time of need.

God gave her the miracle she needed, even if it wasn't the one I wanted for her. I am grateful that I finally got the chance to understand.

BERNIE'S REFLECTION

Life's difficulties are what teach us to grow
as human beings.

Sometimes we are so focused on what we want, we forget the amazing gifts we have already been given. When someone we love is facing cancer, our ultimate goal is their survival. As Jennifer points out, nothing else is acceptable. We want our friends and loved ones to live the long and happy lives they deserve. Unfortunately, it does not always work out that way. However, don't let your anger prevent you from seeing life's real miracles. Miracles come in many shapes and sizes, and doctors would see them more often if they could understand there is no false hope and help people to take on the challenge, not focus on guilt and shame and blame. What is most important is that their lives are still full of happiness and joy; that they get the care, love, and support they deserve.

The books that Jennifer, Laura, and Jamie wrote gave Laura the financial support she needed to spend more time with her family. At the same time, these books provided emotional support for those seeking a little inspiration. What makes our actions meaningful and allows miracles to occur is the response we show to the person with the disease. Jennifer hoped Laura's involvement with the books would grant her friend a miracle of her own. It took a while, but Jennifer came to realize Laura's involvement in the project was the miracle. It takes courage for people to see how a tough situation can be viewed as a blessing, how pain, loss, or illness can be turned around to help heal the world. What Laura has left behind for readers, and most importantly her friends, is the miraculous gift of love and encouragement.

Jennifer finishes her story showing us the only path to immortality: love. It is the only thing of permanence and it lives on after our bodies perish. Thornton Wilder's words from his book *The Bridge of San Luis Rey* say it all: "There is a land of the living and a land of the dying and the bridge is love, the only survival, the only meaning."

The Art of Living

Jane Goldman

I slashed with wild abandon, the crimson stain spread—but not far enough. I drove my knife to its pristine white target, again and again. "So this is what my life's come to," I thought. "At fifty-five, I've become a killer painter."

I've hung my work in galleries and restaurants all over Los Angeles and San Francisco, as well as in Sacramento, California's capital and my adopted hometown of some thirty years. But it's been a long journey to get to the place where I can allow myself to pursue a career in art.

To use a weird old expression, art has always been the elephant in the room for me—seen but not talked about. I've always loved seeing it, touching it, appreciating it, even coveting it. But it's taken me nearly six decades to realize that of the many careers I've enjoyed—from journalism to arts management, TV news to public relations—being an artist is the most fulfilling, joyful, and truly me. It's been more of a midlife epiphany than a crisis: discovering that the ability to succeed and make money doing something is not the same as loving to do that thing.

Although my love for art was born in the great American Midwest—as was I in 1950—it took my migrating west to free my spirit
and hands to begin to actually make some.

I had started my journey in college, when I escaped my tiny
hometown of LaSalle, Illinois (population 10,000), lamming out
for the gallery and museum action of Chicago. There I was able
to explore "real" art as I pursued a bachelor's degree in journalism,
then a career in arts management.

When I moved to California in 1976, the initial goal was to try
my hand at television news. I spent two years as a reporter/anchor
at the local NBC outlet in Sacramento, doing what I'd imagined
would be my "dream job." But I soon met (and married) the man
of my dreams, and left the self-absorbed world of television, mainly
so our work and home schedules would match. But it wasn't until
I turned thirty-five that I began to realize my real calling, when I sat
in on a Life Painting course at Sacramento State University.

As I leaned my seven-months-pregnant belly in the general
proximity of a three-by-three-foot piece of gessoed craft paper
on the floor—my brush going as fast as it could since I knew the
model would change her position in only five minutes—I heard
the teacher, a renowned painter himself, tear my previous work to
shreds. His comments weren't unkind, simply indicative of someone who thought I needed to "learn to see like an artist."

I guess by the end of the class, I was seeing twenty/twenty. After
my husband, Ed, urged me to frame twenty-five of those quickly
rendered figure paintings, a local restaurant asked to display them.
It was my first solo show—and to my astonishment, it sold out. It
was an auspicious beginning. But if I'd thought moving west was a
journey, I hadn't seen nothin' yet.

I'd always prided myself on making my own way, from working
Saturdays during high school and part-time all through college to
earn my tuition, to vying back and forth with Ed over which one of
us was earning more money that year.

The money I began to make selling my paintings was hardly
enough to live on. My output wasn't huge, either, since the only time
I painted was during our baby's naps. It was Ed's turn to make more
that year and for the next several years, while I stayed home with
our new daughter. But the more time I spent with Jessica, the more

whimsical my art subjects became and the less I needed to have something in front of me to create an intriguing composition.

One piece, called "Grandma Babysits," came straight from my own childhood memories, by way of the Twilight Zone. Against a background of perfectly rounded blue trees, a garden of skulls, and two houses (one with flames consuming a clock on the mantel and another with a devil peeking out the window), a woman stood screaming, her hands raised as she looked anxiously toward the figure of a young girl stretched out on a couch, floating in the sky.

My own grandmother did babysit for me one New Year's Eve. As I cried my good-byes, my mother called cheerily, "We'll see you next year!" leaving me to spend the night on Grandma's scratchy mohair couch as an antique clock dinged each hour. I was awake until my parents picked me up in the morning—far sooner than the one-year wait that I'd imagined. Meanwhile my Uncle Rudy, who lived between Grandma's home and ours, used to dress up as a devil every Halloween and run around and around our house to scare my sister and me. And Grandma Spelich did work a large garden until she broke a hip at age ninety-one. All of this combined in my brain and came out on the canvas—how, I'll never know. But a winery owner and art collector from San Francisco loved "Grandma Babysits" as much as I did (and the judges at the State Fair, who gave it top honors) and bought the piece.

That same year, Jessica entered kindergarten and I hit the Big 4-0. I was somehow moved to make a greater contribution to our family bottom line, even though Ed offered to be the solo breadwinner and encouraged me to make art full-time. I went to work for the local utility district, hated that, then joined him in his growing public relations firm, contenting myself to being a weekend painter at most.

Then in 1998, all hell broke loose. I was diagnosed with breast cancer, a particularly virulent form that required one breast to be removed and involved one lymph node. I suspected I was in for a long haul. Lacking the energy for full-time employment, I began painting in earnest during my recovery.

Faced with the harsh reality that my future was far from guaranteed, I began to appreciate the value of stopping to smell—and paint—the flowers. Since it's difficult to contemplate nature without becoming happier, I felt that these flowers had the power to comfort those who viewed them. I began a series called "Power Flowers" that debuted at a local gallery and quickly became the subject of local magazine and newspaper coverage.

The idea that these paintings were a critical step to healing resonated with many women, and my art was featured in a PBS special about breast cancer. The power of flowers was everywhere!

I'd like to tell you that cancer is behind me, but it isn't true. The cancer has recurred just about every year—in the liver, the uterus, the brain, the bones, the other breast, the abdomen, the brain again—each time requiring another dose of chemotherapy and/or radiation, each time turning our lives upside down as we deal with side effects and endless doctor and hospital visits.

When our daughter, Jessica, left for her first year of college, it was as devastating as all my sage women friends had predicted. Even though she hadn't been home that many evenings during her junior and senior years of high school—thanks to a burgeoning acting career—we'd brushed our teeth and washed our faces together and she'd slept in her own bed every night. Being alone during the day wasn't new for me, but it was different knowing Jessica wouldn't be bursting in the door any minute, her beautiful face flushed with the excitement of teenage life. Again, I took solace in making art.

Now, as I wait for her daily phone calls from college instead of her wake-up cries on the baby monitor, I am able to paint for many more hours each day. Ed, who's already been simply the best husband and caretaker anyone could wish for, reminds me daily that my life is mine to live, however I see fit. He's kept his business going at an even stronger pace—and I've been able to at last pursue my dream of a full-time career making art.

I still haven't gotten used to the fact that Jessica is away at school, but my days are different now—in a good way, just as hers are. I get up every morning happy to greet the day. It doesn't matter if I feel nauseous and a bit too tired to lift my head off the pillow. I throw off the quilt, jump (okay, crawl fast) out of bed, and smile as I pass my studio/office on the way downstairs for breakfast. Though I know it can be interrupted at any time by medical trials and tribulations, I find myself welcoming each day knowing that I will fill it doing exactly what I want to do.

I now think of myself as an artist and businesswoman, not some housewife who occasionally makes art. I'm introduced to people who recognize my name and are familiar with my work. I'm not just Mrs. Ed. It's all happened gradually, accompanied by tough challenges. But I've come to think of the cancer as a chronic disease that needs maintenance, like diabetes or heart disease—and to think of painting as some of the best medicine.

I now get together with a handful of other women artists every Wednesday evening for a few hours of making sculpture from porcelain clay that's then fired and either glazed or painted with oils. My first piece in this class, led by the wise and talented Miriam Davis, was of a seminude woman (okay, she wears a thong) seated, fondling her long, curly hair. It's called "Hair Peace" and captures what I feel each time my hair comes back after another session of chemotherapy.

I don't really want to be a poster child for breast cancer, and don't make it a habit to link my art to my illness. Not only have I branched out into landscapes, but I find myself drawn to whimsical subjects again. I just finished a trio of clay mouse-head masks for a group show and then let loose with a sculpture I call "Pillocchio." It's a clay bust of everyone's favorite Disney puppet, complete with jaunty feathered cap and cute little collared shirt. His nose, grown two feet long thanks to his lying, is made of prescription pill bottles I've collected from my pharmacy over the last eight years.

I've realized there's no separating art from illness, it's who I am and what I'm going through that translates into my art. As mature women, we take who we are and go from there. I'm not afraid to let my feelings show in terms of what I create. A killer painter, on the most wanted list at last.

BERNIE'S REFLECTION

Reconnect with your inner artist and create your
unique self-portrait.

The best way to cope with cancer is the way Jane did, to keep living your life with joy, because when you live in your heart,

magic happens. The healthiest state one can achieve is to do
something that makes you lose track of time, and that is exactly
what art can do for you. I've felt it many times myself when
painting. You can achieve a peaceful state of mind, similar to a
trance state, by doing a relaxing activity that can be an outlet for
your feelings as well. Jane found her voice in her art and used
her paintings as a way of expressing things that cannot always
be put into words. By sharing her art with others, she connected
with thousands of other people who know what it feels like to
run their fingers through their hair that has just grown back, or
learned the importance of stopping to smell the flowers, as she
says. Jane's husband's love, acceptance, and encouragement also
helped her to live the life she dreamed of.

There is no separating life from art. Art can help you discover
who you really are and to see the things around you more clearly.
So paint, draw, sculpt, or do whatever you can to tap into your
creative energy during this time. Take up one of the hobbies you
have always put on hold or dreamed of doing. The important
thing is to find a healthy way of expressing yourself. When you
see yourself as a blank canvas and a work in progress, you stop
blaming yourself and feeling guilty. Any artist knows that you
must keep remolding the clay, or repainting the canvas as you see
the world more clearly. So become that work of art and create
your true self.

PART THREE

Healing

Animals as Healers

Jack Stephens

After an all-day board meeting, I was ready to go home. My fellow board members followed me, invited as dinner guests. As soon as I walked into the house, the smell of roast, garlic, and wine lured me into the kitchen, where my wife stood, cooking the evening meal. I gave her a kiss, asking if there was anything that I could do to help. Before she could respond, I noticed a pet carrier sitting on the kitchen floor with a small puppy inside. Although she had a smile on her face, the look in her eyes sensed the inevitable tension she expected to get from me. I was livid, but she knew that I wouldn't start anything right then with company over. My only comment to her was, "You need to take the puppy back." Of course, my dinner guests sided with my wife, encouraging me to keep the puppy. I really didn't need one more responsibility or stress in my life right then. We already had two labs that required our care and attention, and my business as a veterinarian was creating a lot of stress with time away from home.

An early riser, the next morning I was up before the rest of the family. I had nearly forgotten about the puppy when a whimper from the crate sitting next to the bed reminded me of my wife's "gift." I let the puppy out of his crate, took him outside, and then sat down to read the paper as I usually do. What was not usual was the persistent tugging and pulling by this puppy on my socks, which were of course attached to my feet. I continued to read, figuring the puppy would soon lose interest. Rather, he moved on to chewing and tearing at my newspaper, which was of course still in my hands. Unable to keep a smile from creeping across my face, I gave him my full attention. About this time my wife and daughter descended the stairs to witness this nuisance of a dog. "So," I asked in a playful way, "when are you taking Spanky back?" I'd named the puppy, and my wife knew that this was my way of saying that we could keep him, without really having to say the words. She smiled at me and continued into the kitchen for her morning cup of coffee. I knew I shouldn't have been such a hardass.

Spanky immediately became the dominant dog in the house over the two labs, Remington and Brook. Our nightly walk to the park, one block away, became a ritual that they looked forward to. Spanky insisted on the lead position, establishing his dominance. Once at the park, I would throw the ball for the labs in a never-ending game of fetch as Spanky recklessly chased and yelped after them, trying to catch up and steal the ball. Great fun, but our nightly ritual was about to change.

Five months after my wife brought Spanky home, I was diagnosed with stage IV throat cancer, even though I had never smoked. I was given only six to twelve months to live, and the doctor recommended that I take this time off from work. Quit work? Being a vet was one of the most important parts of my daily life, and I couldn't see myself stopping. I enjoyed the daily interactions with the animals and the people. During my treatment I would need this distraction, so I continued to work.

The distraction that I didn't anticipate was Spanky. He seemed to sense more about my condition and mood than any human possibly could. My wife noticed before I did the bond that Spanky and I shared. One night I parked the car in the driveway, walked to the front door, and stepped into the house to find my wife standing at the door waiting for me. She held out a fresh drink, iced and ready.

"How did you know when I would be home? Did someone call and tell you I was on my way?" I asked.

"No," my wife replied, "Spanky let me know you were home, just as he does every night, his usual routine."

"What are you talking about" I asked.

"About five minutes before you arrive, he runs upstairs into the den, sits on the backrest of the couch, and looks out the window and down the street until he sees your car. Then he runs downstairs and sits in front of the door till you walk in," she replied.

Spanky, as usual, hopped around at my feet, wagging his tail, wondering why I hadn't picked him up. I didn't believe my wife, looking from her with that drink in her outstretched hand to Spanky running around at my feet. I just stood there. This was surely a coincidence, so I needed proof. Experimenting with various days and times, we tested this theory and discovered that it worked about 90 percent of the time. Our only response was to laugh.

Spanky's behavior was unexplainable to me. What also disturbed me were my own feelings and connections to Spanky, something I have never felt toward a pet before. Since I was a child, I'd had pets ranging from the usual dogs, cats, and goats to the more unusual pets such as pigeons and even an owl. As a vet, I was trained to heal and make these animals well, yet I found myself in unfamiliar territory.

This connection to Spanky helped explain some questions that had been unanswered during the course of my career as a vet. Some pet owners, I felt, had an attachment to their animals that was excessive. By this I mean, the actual discussions that would take place between pet and pet owner, the lavish leashes and collars combined with the clothing adorned on their pets resembling something that a human would wear: little coats and sweaters, tiny hats and socks, even shoes. But with Spanky, I was beginning to see and feel their level of attachment.

I started to notice other things more closely as well. During treatments at the hospital, I would meet the same patients on a regular basis. Some seemed less ill and had no worse a prognosis, but they did not survive cancer. I wondered what made the difference, but kept coming back to the thought of Spanky. He had the charm to distract me from the awful times, to make me laugh when I didn't feel like laughing, allowing me those moments to forget about the debilitating effects of my treatments. I knew there had to be something more than just an emotional attachment to Spanky, something that required research, an explanation.

My intrigue and interest in this research wore off a little as my treatment progressed; there were nights when I just couldn't find the energy or inclination to take the dogs for their evening walk to the park. Spanky sensed my exhaustion on those nights and sat quietly with me on the couch. Other times, I had only lost my momentum and motivation to go, even though I knew that I would feel better if I went. If my wife would have insisted that I take a walk, I likely would have snapped at her. Yet Spanky sensed that I only needed a little motivation. One night as I sat on the couch, a garbled bark distracted my attention from the television. I looked down to see Spanky standing at my feet. His leash was gently draped in the folds of his mouth as a smile nearly crept over the bulge of his lips, his tail wagging incessantly. He wasn't asking, he was insisting that I get up and go outside with him. I couldn't possibly refuse.

His leash and smile trick didn't work every time, but that didn't stop him from trying a new approach. Although Spanky was a miniature pinscher, he took on the persona of a Jack Russell terrier one night as he began to jump relentlessly in front of the door, from floor to doorknob, over and over again. If he didn't get our full attention with these antics, he would incorporate a bark with each jump. Selfishly, my wife and I would enjoy the spectacle for some time before I ended his suffering and took him for his well-deserved walk.

Over the course of many months, my treatments came to an end and my cancer was officially in remission. My life settled down, becoming more routine; part of this routine included household chores such as mowing the lawn. On a Saturday morning I left Spanky inside as usual, since I would be mowing the front lawn. Somehow, Spanky managed to escape out the back door and, distracted by the mowing, I didn't realize he was out. Cars would come and go without my noticing, but somehow a truck distracted me from my chore. I stopped and watched it drive by, and it was then, after it had passed, that I noticed Spanky lying in the middle of the road. The truck hadn't bothered to slow down or stop. My constant companion was dead. There was nothing that I could do but mourn.

Life had other plans for me, though. The following Saturday, the woman who bred Spanky showed up on my front doorstep, having driven seventy-five miles to my house. As I opened the door, she promptly plopped a puppy resembling Spanky into my arms. I tried to hand the puppy back to her just as quickly: "I don't want another dog. It would not be fair to Spanky." Refusing to take back the puppy, she began walking away. "I am on my way to San Diego. Just keep her for me for the day and I will pick her up on my way home." I don't think I need to bother telling you that she didn't return that day for the dog. By the end of that first hour, I named her Skeeter.

Although Skeeter looks like Spanky, she is shy and timid, content to be a sissy lapdog, where Spanky was bold and outgoing, content only when exploring. I owe a great deal to Spanky. He taught me the true nature and healing power of our relationship with our pets. Through my own exploring, I discovered research validating my suspicions about the benefit of Spanky in my struggle with cancer. Through my own boldness, I founded the Skeeter Foundation, a nonprofit organization to support and educate the public about our beliefs about the human-animal bond and its effects on healing.

Through my own outgoing nature, I am now able to better understand the pet owners who once slightly irritated me with their overindulgences. I am proud to say I've bought Skeeter a fine collection of jackets and sweaters, leashes and collars.

I wake before the alarm clock sounds and sit on the edge of my bed. I look over at my wife and listen to the repetitive rhythm of her breathing, signaling that she is still asleep. Skeeter jumps down from the bed, runs to the bedroom door, and patiently waits for me to let her out. My pillow still holds the imprint from where she slept. I turn off the alarm clock before it sounds, then gently touch the bronze, square box next to it that holds Spanky's remains. Thank you, my friend.

BERNIE'S REFLECTION

Animals are our teachers because they do not need all the
time we do to learn about love and forgiveness.

Before discussing the specifics of Jack's story, let me share that
there are scientifically proven benefits to owning a pet. In one
study, people who owned a dog, after returning home from the
hospital after a heart attack, had a mortality rate at twelve months
of only 5 percent. Those who went home to a house with no dog
showed a mortality rate of 26 percent. When you pet a dog, your
oxytocin and serotonin levels rise. These are the same bonding
hormones that rise after a woman gives birth. So pets help us stay
connected. It is this sense of connection and love that improves
our survival rate and makes it hard not to come home from the
animal shelter with a rescued dog or cat.

Animals live this connection and know how to have their
needs met. They move, make noise, and express feelings, and
Spanky was a perfect example. He was not a submissive sufferer,
he displayed survivor behavior. He showed up with a leap and
a leash and made sure his needs were met. One of our dogs,
Furphy, should have been a lawyer. He never stops telling me
what to do, where to drive, when to feed him, and more. One
time when I was driving, the car was very quiet so I turned to the
backseat to see what he was doing. Turns out I had driven off
with our other dog, Buddy, but not Furphy. So I went home, and
found him in the driveway with a look that told me where I rated
on his list of intelligent people.

Animals can live with a sense of peace that we have a great
deal of trouble achieving. They seem to know beyond a doubt
that we are here to love and our bodies are simply the mechanism
we use to do this. Animals do not need perfect health or bodies
to love and be loved. Thus they can accept their limitations and
afflictions far better than humans can.

Animals also have no trouble finding meaning in their daily
lives and activities. People, on the other hand, find it a problem.
We all need to realize that work is a way to form connections and

relationships. It is about the people we interact with who make our lives meaningful, but unfortunately many people would say they only create trouble. Thank God Jack did not listen to his doctor and quit the work that was so meaningful and fulfilling for him. If you lose the meaning in your life, it can be hard to survive. I had a man walk into my office one day and say, "There's no reason for me to live. I can't work anymore." I pointed out that his wife and two children might be a reason. He looked like I had just hit him on the head with a mallet.

Jack kept a good attitude and listened to his heart wisdom. He had the courage and was brave enough to follow what his heart told him. He stayed with his work and accepted the dog because he felt better when he was with him. Men need to be willing to be aware of their feminine side and their feelings. Dogs make great role models for that, too.

Animals live in the moment, and because consciousness is nonlocal, they can sense the well-being of their owners and predict and warn their owners about impending seizures, heart attacks, skin cancers, and more. We have that ability, too. I could sense in my patients who was doing well and who wasn't. It was like an energy they did or did not radiate when they came into the office. What keeps us from accomplishing this as easily as the animals is that we think too much. I know when I want to communicate with our pets, I must calm down and go into their minds and be with them rather than wondering where are they, why did they do this, and so on. When I do that, it works.

As I have said, life is a series of beginnings. Each time you experience a loss, you must begin again. When Jack lost his dog, he was wise enough to give the new dog another name. He responded to his pain and allowed something nourishing to come from it. Jack's way of using his cancer to find hope and joy was to start the Skeeter Foundation to help educate pet owners. I can tell you that Spanky is proud of his human parents for what they have done. He realizes that because of him, his owners' behavior is almost as good as a dog's.

Grayed Waters

Beverly Hoffman

You must seek the Whale song within you. In hearing Whale's call you will connect to the Ancients on a cellular level.

—Jamie Sams and David Carson

Looking back twelve years ago, my first memory after my biopsy was of my doctor walking into my hospital room, the smell of antiseptic hanging in suspension around her. My senses became more alert, the same way they do on Halloween night when I see blinking pumpkin earrings dangling on a trick-or-treater with green hair. My doctor didn't look up into my eyes. So I knew.

She opted to busy herself paging through my chart, her thumb pushing up on papers condensed with information about me—my age, weight, blood test results, and biopsy report. Then she closed the metal cover, the color of October's night clouds masking the moon. She tapped my chart with her forefinger, a thud that died before she tapped again.

Time spooked me, a howl of thoughts jumbled through my head: "I can't die. They'll fix me, like they did Mom. And Karen. The doctor had said she was certain it wasn't cancer after the needle aspiration."

Time had been an especially dear friend the last month. After I turned in my retirement papers, Time and I dreamed gauzy dreams. We planned months into the future—whether I'd try watercolors or oils. Writing as a second career? And the first place we'd visit—Alaska or possibly the more distant Mongolia? I asked Time what kind of grandparents we'd be.

One night, between sleeplessness and sleep, I turned over and my hand skimmed my breast. A lump? I willed my hand to return to the spot to feel smooth skin—no lump. Then I could dismiss the dark idea that had forced acid into my throat and think only of my dreams for the garden I'd tend. My fingers searched my breast. I found it. *It can't be. Not now. I've waded through grading stacks of essays to enjoy these next sweet years.* I said nothing to my husband that night. Denial is easy. I awoke several times during the night, my hand returning to the spot where instinct, much more accurate than a global positioning system, guided me.

A lumpectomy confirmed cancer. I opted to travel from Panama, where I was a Department of Defense high school English teacher, to Houston. The staff at M.D. Anderson awaited me and thousands of others who traveled from foreign countries each year for a pilgrimage to the Holy Land of state-of-the-art healing, the place that held out a hand of hope. Time compressed as I left lesson plans, told friends, and figured out where to stay for nine weeks in a city I'd known previously only for its humidity and its oil.

Time stuck close to me, ticking its jarring, insistent rhythm. As I was splayed and naked on the radiation table—blue markings indicating the outer bounds and red marks the exact targets— the seconds seemed long enough for me to learn a new language, a complicated and complex language that would take years to learn.

I became part of the process of beating Time. When the radiation strobe searched my body and then aimed at the killer, I waited for its mission to be complete: to obliterate, to keep cancer cells from splitting at rapid-fire pace, lusty to feed on healthy cells, their food of choice, so they could grow into aggressive chow hounds, never satisfied, always hungry. Always searching for one more healthy bite.

I vowed I'd not turn inward and fixate on cancer. My first day at the hospital, I had volunteered for two hours every day helping the staff and patients. After my treatment and my work, I left the smell of Pine-Sol, the wheezing portable oxygen machines, the yellowing skeletal patients with hospital-supplied paisley scarves tied turban-style around their heads, and drove to the three-story Galleria Mall, where safety and the comfort of air-conditioning allowed me the luxury of exercise. I walked for at least an hour.

I had my routine. First, lunch of warm tomato basil soup at a French restaurant that opened onto the ice skating rink. I sipped my soup and watched the skaters glide to music and always tensed my shoulders when their blades braked against the frozen ice with a hollow scraping.

Then, after lunch, I walked. And, of course, considered my future. *Was cancer going to kill me?* At several of the flagship stores' cosmetic counters, I sprinkled myself with quick sprays of Eternity perfume. I inhaled the sweet everlasting fragrance dabbed on my wrists and behind my ears while I kept up my pace.

Finally, I went to the home I would use for nine weeks, the house of a shirt-tail relative, Eulah, in the beginning throes of Alzheimer's. I listened to the same stories several times every night. I finally decided to put them on paper, along with hundreds of her photos dating back to the late 1930s that she'd never organized. I made scrapbooks for her, five of them for close relatives of hers. She housed me and each morning fortified me with fried eggs in butter and bacon. We were a fabulous duo, each of us turning routines into rituals that helped us cope. It took two days to fall in love with Eulah because of her generous heart and the grace she carried as she watched her mind collapse.

At the radiation clinics, my appointments coincided with those of a young man from Mexico who had throat cancer and whose mother's eyes willed him to get well, and with Brooke, a two-year-old, there with her mother, Danielle, and her father, when he got time off. We became a family and shared our journeys of surviving both cancer and Houston juggernauted with traffic. We traded names of restaurants. Of events. Agreed that the new nurse with eyebrows like lions' manes was much too gruff.

Day in and day out, time recycled itself, droning on between scheduled appointments, visits with the doctors, and countless trips up and down hospital elevators with the ever-ringing bell and steel doors that gasped each time they opened. We all waited for the day when we'd get our final booster shot and be on our way. My day was August 1. By then my husband had come up from Panama, after having closed three schools and officially retiring. Together we hurried through the final treatment, and hugged good-bye to the staff and doctors.

We flew to Seattle and drove out to Sequim, our new home. It was our first house, because we had lived in government quarters for almost thirty years, and I asked my husband to carry me over the threshold. How could a special husband deny me that request? He held his breath and lifted me up. We went into our first home. Together. No furniture, of course, but we had plenty of space to dream of our new life.

Time passed, and one by one I marked off five calendar years. I gardened and painted. I chose watercolors rather than oils. Watercolors were more unpredictable and were transparent on the paper. I decorated our house. Washington air filled me with new energy. I walked and memorized poetry.

One particular afternoon I was calf-deep in mud, creating a new garden, thinking of the fact that I had survived without a recurrence of cancer for over five years, that magic number where insurance companies consider cancer patients to be well. I wondered about Brooke, the two-year-old who was to find out whether her cancerous eye had to be removed. I had left the day before the family was to get the verdict. Five years later, I had a strong sense to go inside and call Danielle and see if her daughter had survived and how she was doing. Shovel in hand, seeds to plant, I argued with myself to finish the garden first, and then would call. Time's metallic edge mocked me and taunted me until I took off my shoes, sloshed with mud, and my wet garden gloves. I trudged inside.

When I called Danielle, her sister Tiffany, by chance, was walking through Danielle's house to retrieve a forgotten bag. I told her my story, and she assured me her now seven-year-old niece Brooke was alive and feisty. She promised to relay my message to Danielle, who'd return my call in minutes. I sat in my sunporch, sixty feet above the Strait of Juan de Fuca. The Canadian Rockies hovered deep at the horizon's edge, purple and hazy. The waters of the Strait stretched toward the shore, an incoming tide so gentle, I could see rocks beneath the waves.

The phone rang. Danielle. I sat in an easy chair, looking out in the Strait, as we caught up with one another. Suddenly the waters darkened. I looked into the sky to see if storm clouds were forming. The sky was blue. I looked back at the water. I saw something that I had never seen before and have never seen since. Two gray whales surfaced in unison and then dropped below the water again. After about thirty seconds I saw them surface again and then I lost sight of them.

"Danielle," I whispered. "You'll never believe what I'm seeing. Two whales passing by. Two magnificent grays."

"You're kidding!"

"I'm not." I began crying, touched by Nature's gracious omen of good. In Native American lore, whales are the record keepers. My heart slowed its rhythm to a shaman's drumbeat, the universal heartbeat that aligns all beings heart to heart.

Great lives still to be lived. Brooke's and mine.

Time hugged me as it stretched its arms into the future.

BERNIE'S REFLECTION

*Take time for the simple things, for they are the most
precious.*

I hope as you read Beverly's story that you came to realize the importance of spending your time doing what *feels* good and makes you happy. When you do what brings you joy, you become an active participant in your health.

Sometimes the things that affect survival are very simple, like taking a walk. When you walk, you have the opportunity to become aware of your thoughts and feelings and not be distracted by the meaningless nonsense most people are involved in. Studies have shown that walking can be more therapeutic than taking an exercise class. I feel it is because your thoughts become more focused while walking by yourself versus the activities carried out in a class.

The other survival activity that Beverly displayed was her willingness to help others out of a genuine desire to do so, and at the same time, not deny her needs and feelings. When you give love, you benefit. Volunteers live longer, happier lives when the act of volunteering is coming from a genuine desire to help others and not about guilt or a denial of your own needs.

As a painter I know how meaningful creating a work of art can be. When the activity you are involved in makes you lose track of time, it takes you away from your daily world and cares; it is like being in a healthy meditative state. I consider this to be the healthiest state anyone can be in. It gives your body a positive message, and whether it is gardening, painting, or playing with your grandchildren, it is healing time for you.

Last but not least is the therapeutic effect of nature. In a hospital room or an apartment, those who can see nature through the window experience less pain and stress than those who are on the first floor looking out at a brick wall. Think about Beverly's reaction to seeing the whales. She took them as a sign from God that she would survive. When you become one with the wonder of nature, anything is possible. She calls it a gracious omen of good, and literally that is what creates true healing and miracles.

Chinese Finger Trap

Judith Fraser

W here've you been?" George, an acquaintance at my neighborhood gym, asked as he stepped onto the treadmill next to mine. "You've been gone for at least six months." Since I'd always felt comfortable sharing bits of my life with him in the past, I answered truthfully, "I had cancer. But, now I'm okay." Actually I was moving slower than usual, but just to be up and out of bed seemed like a huge improvement over what I'd gone through. The operation plus six weeks of radiation had left me feeling like a rag doll with some of her stuffing pulled out.

I glanced out the windows that stretched across the gym to our right. The autumn wind blew some of the multicolored leaves from the nearby trees against the glass. They made a gentle crinkling sound—reminding me that the season was once again changing. Time was moving on and I was still very much a part of it.

George tilted his black cap down over his dark eyes to block out some of the glare from the sunlight. "Well, what did you do to cause that?" he said in a low, even monotone.

What had he just said? My stomach tensed as his words exploded in my head. What had I done to cause that? My fingers gripped harder around the handrail of my treadmill to steady my legs. I forced my breath to go deeper into my diaphragm in order to calm the zigzagging of my heart.

His question was startling. I'd shared something vulnerable about myself, and I expected my friend to say something encouraging in return. Something like the words I'd heard from so many well-wishers lately that would have felt good—"Well, looks like you made it through a difficult passage," or "Sorry you had to go through that." Instead, his words—sounding direct and all-knowing—shook me to the core.

George was making me look at my shadow side, the part of me that in the past had felt secure in the false belief that I was in control of my life. The arrogant, innocent part that thought I was above such a serious illness as cancer. Never mind that 90 percent of my relatives had died from cancer, I'd willed myself past their genetic weakness. I ate the right vegetables, fruits, and fish. I took vitamins, exercised (look—there I was at the gym right at that very moment), meditated on a daily basis, and even taught stress reduction to hundreds of overstressed people. My head was on straight and my feet were on the ground. Cancer was all a matter of the weak-willed, right? And I wasn't weak, ever.

Pictures of myself sitting in my doctor's office danced across the inside of my head as I continued walking on the treadmill.

I'd gone in to see him because my stomach hurt. The pain had been persistent and no matter what I did, it wouldn't go away.

After my examination, he stood in front of me, glanced down at his chart then up into my eyes. "You have cancer," he said as gently as he could.

"Cancer?" I questioned. I could feel my forehead tensing into thin, squiggly frown lines. "No." I shook my head. "There must be some mistake, all I have is a stomachache."

His eyes softened. I'm sure I wasn't the first one to question his diagnosis. "It's definitely cancer," he said. "And, it's advanced."

Stunned and shaken, I felt like I was in the middle of a seven-point earthquake. The world went fuzzy. For a few minutes I wasn't sure where I was, or who I was. Did he say the "C" word? He must be wrong. Maybe he has the wrong Judith Fraser? Or the wrong report? In a second, he'll notice his mistake, and it will all be another glitch in my past. I pulled on the cloak of denial as easily as a child pulls on a Superman or princess cape.

My thoughts cleared. This was real, and I managed to ask: "What's my next step?" Even in that frail state, I wanted some control over something.

"A CAT scan." The doctor answered. CAT scan? A recent dream I'd had suddenly became quite clear. I was on an ocean liner. I tried to save a cat perched on the edge of a railing. And failed. The cat bit me on the back of the neck. It was my unconscious trying to alert me to my body's need for modern machinery.

After my operation, the doctor announced, "The cancer in your uterus was unusual. It was a sarcoma and could have grown anywhere in your body. You were fortunate that it grew in an area that is protected." The doctor looked down at his chart, then added, "You also had another kind of cancer in your cervix that we've cauterized."

Another dream suddenly became clear. There was a large pool of water with a guitar case submerged in the center on my patio. I fretted that the guitar inside would be ruined. The delicate strings and smooth casing would no longer be able to send music into the world.

Over to one side of the pool was a broken pot filled with small flowers. I worried that the flowers would die. They were no longer safely contained.

The guitar case in my dream was a perfect image for the protection my body had provided for the sarcoma. It gave me hope and a greater respect for the wisdom of my body than I'd ever had before.

There was second symbol in the dream—the broken flowerpot— it was telling me that my cervix was going to be "deflowered." Wow! That was a lot of information that came from somewhere deep inside of me.

"What alternative treatments have helped cases like mine?" I remember asking the doctor.

"I don't know," he said.

I didn't know it at the time, but looking back, I can see that he really didn't hold out much hope for me. He thought my days were numbered. But then, he wasn't the one having amazing dreams, I was.

At the gym, the leaves continued to make their slight tinkling sound as they hit against the windows nearby. *I Love Lucy* played above our heads on one of the televisions suspended from the ceiling. Several people on various pieces of gym equipment listened to the show on their earphones. George turned his head and lifted his eyebrows. "Well?"

I hadn't answered George. Not because I wanted to be rude, but because I didn't know what to say. My silence seemed to encourage him to go further. "You know we're responsible for everything that happens to us, don't you? I mean, everything that happens to us is of our own doing." Drops of sweat beaded on his deep forehead.

I knew that he wanted to help, but I felt like we were both speaking a different language. I couldn't speak his and I couldn't explain to him what was going on inside me. In fact, I was afraid to tell him what was going on inside me for fear that somehow there would be another judgment that I couldn't face.

"If you'd like, I can help you see what you've done wrong," George said as his chest heaved in and out from the quickness of his steps.

The noise of his words continued to beat against my body like an unsuspected hailstorm as we continued to walk side by side. His workout was set on "random" and included various fast speeds and high inclines. My workout was set at "manual," a slow pace—no inclines. I was not trying to keep up—just trying to move forward.

The cacophony of sounds from exercise machines and various conversations of those around us wove in and out of my self-guilt. I could see Lucy and Desi laughing on the television screen while my mind was busy trying to think through George's question.

"Had I done something to cause my cancer?" I asked myself. Thoughts whirled through the dark cave in my head, searching for somewhere to land that would make sense. Every once in a while they landed on something.

Once it was sadness. My dog had died a few months previously. A friend told me that sadness could weaken the immune system.

The death of my dog was devastating. My heart ached so much, I wanted to take it out and hold it in my hands.

Then food. "You are what you eat," the saying goes. I had to admit that I hadn't always eaten as well as I had done in the past several years. There was a time when I had to have ice cream after dinner. And fried foods used to taste good, a long time ago.

Then again, maybe it wasn't food, maybe it was breathing in too many toxins. I read recently that standing next to the pump when you put gas in your car can cause cancer. And the air—that brown haze that hangs over the city can cause cancer. I can see that haze hovering like a dirty carpet from the mountain ridge above my house.

All the possibilities of what I might have done wrong raced through my head, but I still didn't know what to say to my friend. We continued our side-by-side workout in awkward silence.

At home I continued to ponder George's words. What had I done to cause my illness? *Everything that happens to us is of our own doing.* I'd heard those kinds of statements before, but this time was different. Accepting getting a cold or the flu was different from getting cancer or something that could actually kill me.

After a few days of pondering, I realized that even if I had caused my illness or been responsible for it in some way, the self-blame of those thoughts was stressful. It kept me looking at the past, not the present. It kept me away from seeing the positive of what had occurred. I had gone through a dark passage of the soul, a "hero's journey" of my very own, and emerged on the other side with a bit more wisdom, a lot less expectation, and a deeper respect for my dreams.

I continued drinking my wheat grass juice three times a day. My husband, Ian, had a special set of shelves made for me to grow my own grass. Just running it through my hands made me feel good. And the smell—umm, there's nothing like the fresh scent of healing wheat grass.

My daughter, Tiffany, took me to see her acupuncturist several times a week. Besides strengthening what he called my "kidney" area, he also gave me a small jar of dried ground mushrooms to help my body build more strength to fight off cancer. Even with surgery and radiation, I knew that my cancer could be lurking inside waiting for an opportunity to grow once again. I was to have CAT scans every three months for the next year to give me a chance to fight back as quickly as possible.

Amy, my daughter-in-law, gave me a drawing book complete with colored pencils. I continued to put my feelings—in abstract form—on the white pages of the book. Amy's an artist, so when she draws something, you can tell what it is. When I draw, it's colors and shapes, and no one can tell what it is but me.

My friend Lynne shared her healing tapes with me. I particularly enjoyed the one that took me deep inside a cave in my body. The cave was filled with treasures. Each time I visited the cave, I unearthed new possibilities, golden nuggets of a happy future.

When anything stressful came up, I did the Inner Journey Process I developed with my friend AnnaMay. I would breathe into the stress with awareness by imagining my breath weaving in and out of the dark, wiry webs that stress creates in a caring way. The Journey has helped me to be compassionate with myself in new ways as I let go of judgment about what should and shouldn't be.

It was this process that helped me to reexamine the fear that came up when my friend questioned me about being the cause of my illness. The message I received from that amazing intelligence that lives inside of me was, "Maybe he's right, maybe I caused it. But it doesn't help to examine how or why. Just be compassionate with the cancer. It is the stressor."

I began to examine what I'd kept trying to deny: I had cancer. I may still have cancer. But I turned the negative thought about cancer around.

I began to question my beliefs as well as my friend George's beliefs. What if cancer isn't always bad? What if my cancer was trying to help my body rebalance itself? Questioning in this way brought about a new answer. It was one of those "aha" moments that spring from deep within. It's hard to say the exact words, but in an instant I was given a gift of incredible insight.

I continued to look at cancer as if it was a teacher—trying to help rebalance my body. The effect was amazing. It changed my thinking in so many ways.

The weakness I experienced from my operation and the radiation reminded me to put day-by-day problems in a different perspective. If a dead car battery delayed me in getting to an appointment, it was no big deal. It was just something that, in time, could be taken care of. If I was too tired to meet friends for dinner, it was no big deal. We could have dinner another time. When an electrical shortage cut off all the power in the house, it, too, was no big deal. I knew the power would eventually return to normalcy. Most of the day-to-day problems I experienced while going through my recovery were not life-threatening. They were just little bumps or detours in the road of life.

Many years ago, my children had a toy called a Chinese Finger Trap. It was a small, round cylinder woven out of bark, and when they put their fingers into each end and pulled, their fingers would get stuck. But when they surrendered to the strength of the trap, their fingers were set free. They loved the experience of it. To them, it was magic.

As I continue to search for the positive in problems that come up for me, I think about that trap. When I try to control things that I have no control over, it makes me feel like I'm stuck. When I "let go" and do my Inner Journey Process, I feel the release of stress fall away.

On my recent doctor's visit, I told him that I'd discovered the answer to the question I'd asked him some time before. "The alternative treatment for cancer is love," I said. "Love, of life and of each other." He nodded and smiled.

I know it wasn't technically something he'd studied in medical school. But from the look on his face, I think he agreed.

BERNIE'S REFLECTION

Learn to let go and start living.

Judith learned a lot from her experience, and we can all benefit by learning from her newly gained wisdom. As Judith says, cancer became her teacher. You go into the cave within you to find your treasure and are no longer afraid of the demon guarding it. She became free of blame and willing to learn about life. Suddenly her life was not so distressing and all problems became minor obstacles. Judith no longer sweats the small stuff because, compared to cancer, it's all small stuff.

Control was a big issue and a frequently used word for Judith. As I have said before, our thoughts are the only things we can control. With her "Inner Journey Process," Judith centered her thoughts and feelings. She demonstrated how helpful controlling our own thoughts can be. We can keep things in perspective and remember what is important. This enables us to feel secure and reassures us that things are not as "out of control" as they seem. When you accept, let go, and stop trying to control events, you will find peace, love, and healing, and will derive all their physical, emotional, and spiritual benefits.

I always urge you to respond from your heart when asked, "How are you?" Be sure your response is genuine and your answer is not based on a desire to make others happy. Judith told George, "I'm okay now." Be careful about who you share your life, your feelings, and your information with. George asked his question with a lack of compassion that came from not having experienced cancer himself. He was coming from his head and not his heart. Share your wounds only with those who can listen to you and guide you to a place of inner healing. Usually they are those who have been wounded in some way, too, and can serve out of love. Love is not an alternative therapy. It is a necessity for survival, and there is nothing it cannot cure.

George was not coming from a place of love, and he acted insensitively when he asked in an accusing tone, "Well, what did you do to cause that?" I used to be accused of blaming patients when I would ask them what had happened recently in their life, and how they might be benefiting from their illness. But I am not saying that you caused your illness, nor am I blaming you. However, I am asking you to look at why you might be vulnerable now. The more changes you may have experienced, the more vulnerable you can become to illness. And I am asking you to look at how you can heal your life in order to derive the physical benefits provided by a healed life's internal chemistry.

It's not about blaming yourself for what you did wrong, but about looking at issues like the death of a family member or a beloved pet, the loss of a job, your spouse having an affair, divorce, and more. You can't separate your health from your life and yes, you do affect your life by your decisions. Once again, blame and guilt don't accomplish anything helpful. The question now is, "How can I be loving to myself and create a new life?"

Judith talks about the amazing intelligence dwelling deep within her that was revealed through her dreams and drawings. We need to pay attention to our inner wisdom and the body's ability to communicate through symbols and images. I believe the guitar case in Judith's dream represented her uterus because they have a similar shape and it is where life is created. And though she says her drawings were abstract, she knew they were about her feelings, and the chosen shapes and colors meant something. The therapeutic power of our dreams and drawings unfortunately is not a part of the medical school curriculum. I suggest you try drawing your treatment options and look at them with your family and friends to help you decide what to do.

When you actively participate in your choices around treatment options, you are no longer the "good" patient and submissive sufferer; you become an active and responsible participant in your life. Blame, guilt, and "why?" are no longer issues; life is. Like the Chinese finger trap, when you struggle to win and be free, you remain trapped in its grip. When you let go in order to focus on healing and allow yourself to stop struggling to win the battle, you break free of its grip and start living.

Checkmate

Verna Dreisbach

The freezer door sticks, as usual, and I jerk on the handle one more time with greater force to open it. I reach in for the vanilla ice cream, and the cold mist from the freezer flows like a river out and then down around my feet. My toes curl as the cold penetrates my skin. I grab the cardboard container and slam the door shut. Prying off the lid, I wonder if there is enough for me and my grandfather to share. Whatever might be missing in ice cream, I can make up for with Hershey's chocolate syrup. I scrape the last bit of ice cream out of the container, my hand covered in vanilla from the depths of the carton. Next is the syrup. What artistic creation can I make this time? A happy face with hair? A volcano? A heart? I display the masterpiece to my grandfather, who is seated in his usual chair, and wait for his response. My grandfather looks up from the chessboard, peeking above his reading glasses, as he takes his bowl. He looks at the artwork and smiles. I sit opposite his feet on the floor, my usual spot, bowl in my lap. He has set up the chessboard for our nightly game, each piece in its place, the white on his side, the black on mine. A man of few words, he studies the board and begins to whistle as he makes the first move, a pawn, E3.

You were admitted to the hospital for pneumonia. I don't ever remember you being sick until then. Your cold wouldn't go away and finally you gave in and went to the doctor. It wasn't long before we all knew—advanced lung cancer. I drove to the hospital, determined to see your face, to see in your eyes whether this fate was true. Inside, the room was blinding. Everything appeared white; the floor, the curtains, the bedding, even the daylight shining through the window created the illusion of white, nontransparent glass. As I waited for my eyes to adjust, the faintest wisp of Old Spice filled my nose. Was this you? Family and friends filled the room, and I pushed my way through and stood at the foot of your hospital bed. I don't recall who was there, but they were sad, and some were crying; I only looked at you. I didn't speak or announce my presence. You turned away from those who had your attention and looked directly at me. For a moment, we were the only two people in the room, and silence filled the air with expectation. Your eyes. It was true. How dare you! It was a cancer you could have prevented, didn't you realize the significance of that. I hated those boxes with the damn camel on it. "I hope those cigarettes were worth it." I turned and left.

Only once in a while would we need to consult the guide to determine whether or not a move was legal. Between moves, I stir my vanilla ice cream and syrup into a smooth and creamy blend. I move my pawn, E2.

Our relationship was based upon a mutual understanding and appreciation, one with few words. I knew you best when we laughed together. I wanted to laugh again like we did when I was only four years old and you took apart my See and Say toy, changing the parts around so that when I pulled the string, the arrow landed on the pig, and the sound that came out would be that of a cow. When the arrow landed on a coyote, it would quack like a duck. I wanted that moment back, many of those moments. I wanted those same moments with you for my daughter one day, giving her the same joyful memories I had.

My grandfather, tolerant of my persistent meddling, continues to hum and whistle as he strategically determines his positions on the game board, Bc4, a bishop.

I wanted you to ease my fears about your illness, that I would be all right without you. I learned as a toddler that you had the power to soothe my fears. Not many children learned to walk and ride their bikes in casts from their knee to their toes. What did the doctors know; the crookedness was in my knee, which later resolved itself. When the time came to cut my cast off at the hospital, I was so terrified by the sound and sight of the electric saw that you took me home and slowly cut away the cast yourself with a tiny handsaw.

My legs begin to fall asleep and I have to change positions already. I roll onto my tummy, propped up on my elbows, chin directly above my ice cream bowl. I move a bishop, too, Bc2.

I expected you to be a part of my own family one day, to walk me down the aisle and give me away to a man that I know you would have approved of. I wanted to see your face and tears of joy at the arrival of my first child. Your approval and guidance meant everything to me.

The sound of bluegrass that filled the house stops as the needle reaches the end of the last song. My grandfather gets up from his chair to place another record on the turntable. Music fills the air once more and my grandfather returns, the queen this time, Qf3.

Even with the diagnosis of lung cancer, you continued to laugh, whistle, and work. You continued to play chess with me and eat vanilla ice cream drenched with Hershey's chocolate syrup. Our games did not last as long and I gave you the larger share of the ice cream, but the games didn't matter as much anymore. Somehow they had changed. I didn't care about winning or the strategy, and neither did you. We enjoyed the ritual, the time.

I get up to stretch my legs and place the empty ice cream bowls in the kitchen sink. I can't resist the jar full of chocolate kisses on the counter in front of me. I grab one for me and one for my grandfather and return to our game.

I would have liked to spend more time with you, but I was too busy growing up and starting a career. I assumed that we could spend more time with each other when my life slowed down, after my career was established. That didn't happen. I only came home during the holidays.

I don't want that to happen again. I don't want to get to the end of my life and miss out on my own family—my husband and my children. I don't want to regret missing the play time, creating memories of laughter or witnessing their moments of accomplishment. I didn't have enough experiences, enough memories with you. I wanted more. I needed more. I took for granted one of the most important relationships in my life, even though I have little doubt as to how much we knew we meant to each other.

The chocolate kisses fail to distract him. My grandfather's final move, I wasn't paying attention, the queen, Qxf7, checkmate.

You finished work on Friday and died on Sunday.

Occasionally, I win. My grandfather isn't one to "let" me win. I have to earn my expertise. It is a learning process, not a contest, and I never feel slighted by our games together. This is not a time to talk about the day's activities or about the news, but to sit quietly, concentrate, and enjoy the moment.

Even though I know it is unlikely, I plead for another game. Having already played for an hour or more, he tempts me instead with a lesson on his scientific calculator. I jump up from the floor onto his lap, my face presses against his; a day's worth of stubble scratches my delicate skin and the smell of Old Spice fills my nose. My grandfather knows I view this machine of his with awe and intrigue with the many buttons, symbols, words, and colors, and he enjoys showing me all of its many functions. After dragging out my lesson as long as possible, it is my job to put the chess pieces away and return the game to the cabinet for the following day's challenge.

You taught me the value of family and the importance of having someone to love, trust, and depend upon. Unfortunately, I didn't learn this lesson until after your death, as I took time for granted. This will never happen again. I will be there for my own family; smiling with joy as my husband and I celebrate our vows, holding my daughter's hand to ease her fears in the back of the ambulance, crying for joy when my boys make their first triple play, tucking them in at night and reading them bedtime stories. Time is all that I have.

Your death made me think about time, about family. I became a stay-at-home mom and home-schooled my children. My choices have created a happier, stronger family, not only with me and my husband, but the kids with each other. We are able to spend more family time together, to relax and enjoy our days without the clock ticking away as the days seem to pass us by. My fondest memories are by far the mornings. As the sun rises, the children, one by one, climb into bed and snuggle under the covers until we are all covered in pillows, blankets, cats, and kids. This is our time to cuddle, read, and talk. There is absolutely no better way to wake up in the morning, and I hope that they remember these moments as much as I remember my moments with you. I want my family to know that they are the most important part of my life and that I will always be there for them, to see them every day and cherish every moment. They have no doubt in their minds that I will be home for them, to witness their proudest moments and cherish their deepest feelings, just as you did for me.

I will have to remember our game of chess and any new strategies we discovered. My grandfather never forgets what I have learned and he will be sure to remind me of my error and lack of focus if I fail to apply it. I will find my way to bed, going over the tools I have learned this night. He won't win that way tomorrow. He will have to find himself a new trick!

BERNIE'S REFLECTION

Accept your limited time and spend it with the
people you love.

"Checkmate" is a story that demonstrates the effect that spending true quality time together can have on people. When my wife did stand-up comedy at our presentations, one line she would use that I'm sure you all have heard is, "Life is uncertain. Eat dessert first." So I suggest you enjoy the ice cream and the chess game and live in the moment. Verna's appreciation for the little details has helped her to create vivid memories that will last a lifetime.

Having a grandfather who went above and beyond the call of tenderness helped her to be able to share emotions and create memories that will span generations. Her grandfather will always be present to Verna within her memories.

All relationships evolve over time, often growing into more than either person could have anticipated. Grandparents and grandchildren generally share a bond that transcends traditional language. As Verna says, it is not about the activity, but about the time spent together. Grandparents have the often overlooked luxury of relating like a schoolyard friend while maintaining the respect of a parent. This allows them a chance to influence as a friend might and to teach as someone grand can.

Anger is a part of the five steps of acceptance for a reason: it applies to anything that permanently alters a person's life. Feeling betrayed, Verna became angry with her grandfather for not taking better care of himself, and she blamed him for getting cancer. The fact that Verna took such a normally destructive emotion and used it to make changes for positive results should be commended. Disappointment and anger melted into the realization of how important time with her family really is. She took the blame she initially tried to rest upon the shoulders of her grandfather and looked at life through his eyes. The best memories of Verna's grandfather will still be with her when she plays chess or puts chocolate syrup on her ice cream even years from now.

After that Sunday, the author understood that it was time to reevaluate her life. Remembering the joy of the time spent with her grandfather, she decided to make sure to experience that same bond with her own family. The love for her children gave her the strength to identify the problems in her life and the wisdom not to make the mistakes she felt that she made while growing up. So don't just inform your children, truly educate and inspire them; but most important of all, love them.

Halcyon Days

Andrea Malinsky

O kay, you proved your point.
Life is not all candy and parties.
And long, sunny, warm summer days.
And laughter.

It has been a long, hard, cold winter for too long.
I hate winter.

But at last it's summer again.
And the tears I cried have given birth to new flowers.
And I bask in splendid sunshine.
The gift of light and love and understanding is mine.

I beat you.
You were not stronger.
You tried to be.
But you weren't.
And I am back.
Better than before.

And I will excel.
I will love.
I will see my daughter grow.

I will become powerful again.
I will fly again.
Nobody will be able to reach me.

My halcyon days are finally here.
And they will last forever.

BERNIE'S REFLECTION

When we believe life is good, it becomes good.

The phrase "halcyon days" is a literary commonplace in the English language and culture, signifying the ideals of prosperity, joy, liberation, or tranquillity. The usage derives from the ancient Greek legend of Alcyone. In the legend, the halcyon is a type of kingfisher that builds its nest on the surface of the ocean; the bird charms the winds and waves so that the seas remain unusually calm during its nesting season, the fourteen days preceding the winter solstice.

Andrea's poem is a perfect example of this. She will fly and soar above her problems and survive the winter. She will calm the sea of life and ride out the storms—which we all encounter—so she can survive. Andrea's tears have provided strength and nourishment to her, and she has come to know herself as a survivor who will experience halcyon days. Tears help us to soften the hard, dry, unyielding objects in our lives.

Some of us who have faced our own life or health challenges might write a poem about the turbulent sea of life and the long, hard, cold winter that never seems to end. But Andrea chose to focus on the positive that could come from the experience. Each of us has a choice as to how we define our experience even when we are confronting the same problem and diagnosis.

I know survivors are far more likely to turn their feelings into creative efforts, and writing poetry can be a very healing experience. I wrote many poems during the years when I suffered from the emotional side of being a doctor, for which I was not prepared by my training in medical school. When you write poetry, you get to know yourself, your pain, and your needs. You become aware of and realize that there are some beautiful moments, and they deserve a poem, too.

Finding My Voice

Christine Holmstrom

When I was a little girl, sometimes I'd wake up in the middle of the night, terrified by a recurring nightmare. I couldn't name the frightful thing that woke me; all I could do was jump from my bed and flee to safety. Running through the darkness to my parents' bedroom, I'd cry out: "Mommy! Daddy! I had a bad dream!" And every time, Dad carried me back to my bed, snuggling next to me until I fell asleep. I was safe, the monster banished by his protective presence.

But I'm a grown woman now, and Daddy can't save me from my real-life nightmare—cancer. Somehow, I have to overcome the terrifying monster that dwells inside my own body and calm the frightened little girl that lives in my heart.

When my doctor tells me that the lump in my left breast is probably cancer, I spiral down a vortex of fear. Dark thoughts flood my brain, spilling into my heart and washing away my natural optimism. I exit the medical building like a sleepwalker, my mind swathed in shadow. Even the warmth of the April sun can't penetrate my gloom. My anxiety radiates beyond my body, draining the world of joy. Ordinarily I am charmed by the antics of the little beggar birds that inhabit parking lots, but I barely notice the coterie of sparrows feasting on a discarded roll near my car. My senses are numb to the small pleasures of life.

I stumble through the next few days, feeling doomed and help-less. I am uncertain about the recommended surgery, and averse to undergoing radiation. According to the Western medical model, both are key to eliminating breast cancer, but I resist. My rebellious inner teen demands to know why I can't just heal myself with positive thoughts and natural remedies. I consider that option for a while. However, my distrust of unproven methods propels me toward medically accepted treatments. I am a reluctant patient, though, a victim of this insidious disease and the prescribed treatments.

Two weeks before the scheduled surgery, I sit in my small office, feeling sorry for myself. I know that my negative thoughts won't help me overcome cancer, but my mind won't cooperate. Like a surly child, my brain refuses to budge. The overhead fluo-rescent light flickers as I struggle to focus on a memorandum. Unable to concentrate, I let my thoughts wander. I lean toward the cobalt blue vase on the corner of my desk, inhaling the scent of yellow freesias. The sweet smell awakens me like a dreamer roused by a shaft of morning sunlight, and my fears fade like the night's dreams.

For the first time since the diagnosis, I can think clearly. I recog-nize that I can honor my frightened inner child without letting her rule my life. I decide that my negativity is a bigger enemy than the cancer. Fear is natural in the face of a potentially life-threatening disease, but I can't allow it to paralyze me. I see that I need to take action.

I approach my situation like a puzzle, one piece at a time. First, there's the surgery. "What's my hesitation?" I ask myself. In my heart, I know the answer. I don't have an emotional connection with my surgeon. I require more than skilled hands and medical expertise; I want a warm heart.

I finally see that I have choices. I can forge my own path. It's not only fear that dwells inside, but wisdom and intuition, too. I can listen to my true voice. Thus I begin my journey toward healing.

I decide to seek advice and comfort from the sisterhood of one-breasted women. I phone a colleague who gave a talk on breast cancer to our employee group a few years before. "Find a physician you like," Dawn declares. She recommends Dr. Ernie Bodai, the unstoppable dynamo behind the breast cancer research stamp sold at the post office. I make an appointment for the end of the week.

His office, located on the second floor of the medical center, contains a well-appointed living room, with comfortable couches, inspirational books on the shelves, and lots of boxes of Kleenex. Dr. Bodai greets me with a teddy bear hug and a smile that crinkles the corners of his mouth. "Call me anytime," he proclaims, handing me a card with his pager number. As we sit discussing the provisional diagnosis, he looks directly in my eyes, nodding in understanding. My eyes grow blurry, but I feel comfortable with my tears, not embarrassed. He hands me a tissue and we talk briefly about surgical options—lumpectomy or mastectomy. Dr. Bodai guides me toward the well-stocked resource center to view DVDs that feature interviews and unaltered seminude photos of women who've chosen one of the two options. I am relieved to know what to expect and to discover that I won't face permanent disfigurement no matter what choice I make.

Prior to surgery, I look for ways to prepare my body and mind for what's to come. I try hypnotherapy. I use visualizations and affirmations. I pray. My dear friend Margaret volunteers to take a few vacation days to help care for me after the operation. The fearful ogre of doubt and trepidation has vanished. I am ready.

After surgery, I have a new set of decisions to make. Radiation is the next part of the treatment protocol, but I am hesitant. "Why not use natural remedies and affirmations?" I think again. My inclination is to support my body, not assault it. Yet when I hear the steadfast recommendations of several doctors to undergo radiation, I am filled with doubt. "You will have a 60 percent chance of long-term survival with surgery alone," says Dr. Rosemary, a holistic doctor. "With radiation; the rate rises to over 80 percent." I examine my beliefs—what I really think, not just what I'd like to believe. I don't have the unwavering faith needed to stake my life on alternative medicine alone.

Radiation it is, with a liberal dose of complementary therapies. "If I'm going to jitterbug with jumping atoms," I think, "I'd better have some support." I return to the hypnotist, and call a homeopath who prepares a flower essence formula specifically designed for the victims of the Chernobyl nuclear meltdown. I say any affirmation before each treatment and use vitamin E oil to soothe my increasingly tender breast afterward. Most of all, I rely on humor to dispel any dark thoughts.

The radiation nurses and technicians are upbeat, compassionate, and skilled. "Nothing like being tortured by professionals," I joke with them as I lie on the table, waiting for my radiation treatment. "Zap me good," I laugh.

Now, a decade later, I don't identify with the cancer or the treatments. That part of my life seems like a half-forgotten dream. I am neither a victim nor a survivor.

I sit at my desk, reflecting on my journey. Sometimes, the part of me that is afraid, scared of disease and death, begins its insidious whispering. "What if the cancer recurs? What if it has metastasized? What if you need surgery, radiation, and even chemo?" Like water swirling down a drain, my thoughts are inexorably pulled into a vortex of anxiety. I've learned that I can't ignore or dismiss the voice. I let it speak, and then, like a solicitous parent calming an anxious toddler, I acknowledge, "You are afraid. That's okay. Remember, I love you." I imagine hugging and kissing the little child within. Then I focus on the life around me. I look out the window at the purple fountain grass swaying in the morning breeze, watch a nuthatch teetering at the edge of the courtyard fountain—dipping down for a drink and wiggling his wings in a feather fluffing dance. A chattering squirrel squats on a branch of the big oak, scolding our twenty-pound tabby cat lounging half-asleep on a chair below. I am grateful to be alive, for the beauty and wonder of every day. And I am especially grateful for my inner wise woman, whose voice led me to the path of hope and healing.

BERNIE'S REFLECTION

Choose love, because when you love your enemies,
they cease to exist.

Christine mentions that as a child, she was frequently troubled by nightmares. When you have the courage, at any age, to confront your demons, the nightmares will stop. They are trying to get you to resolve your fears in order to become stronger. When you stop asking, "Why me?" and start asking, "What can I do with this?" your life will change. We all have fears, but when we have the courage to face them, our healing journey begins.

Christine discusses spiraling into a vortex of fear. My wife was diagnosed with breast cancer recently, but because of my experience treating cancer over the past thirty years, we are not in a downward spiral filled with fear. We are living for today and not imagining what could happen. Forty years ago she was diagnosed with multiple sclerosis, and I wasn't mature enough then to not live with the fearful image presented to me by our neurologist. His predictions didn't happen, and part of the reason is that I learned there is more to healing and surviving than doctor's predictions and prescriptions. Christine eventually acted like a survivor and integrated many healers and their remedies into her plan. That was survival behavior.

We must remember that fear can protect us from threats to our lives. It mobilizes our brain and body so that we can flee the demons that threaten us. But if you live in fear, it depletes your ability to resist disease and survive. To grow and heal, one must replace fear with love, hope, faith, and joy, as Christine did, and then your internal chemistry will help you to overcome and survive disease.

Living with negative images and fears is self-defeating. Define your fears so they are not vague and uncertain, and you will see that you are capable of living with them and overcoming them. When someone says, "I'm afraid of dying," I can't help them until I know what that really means. When fear is defined as pain, isolation, or lack of response to their treatment, the person can realize they have the ability to deal with the problems they are confronted with.

Individuals with a survivor personality do not fear failure; they show up and step up to the challenge. They know self-induced healing is possible and is ultimately what we all do. The treatment choices should come from our inner wisdom and intuition that Christine mentions. A patient's dreams can help her become aware of this source of wisdom and lead her to do what is right for her. When you have a dream in which a cat named Miracle walks up to you and tells you what chemotherapy protocol to follow, you know it is coming from a place of knowing. The woman who had the dream discussed it with her doctor, and they followed Miracle's advice, and she is well today. So when in doubt, listen to your heart, dreams, and inner wisdom.

As a surgeon, I have seen the enormous difference in patients' recoveries when they knew I cared about them and saw the surgery as a gift that would help them to be well and survive. This is true of all types of treatment. When you see yourself as being poisoned by chemotherapy and burned by radiation, you are more likely to live out your negative images and expectations. When you see them as gifts from God, you are more likely to heal and to have minor or no side effects. It is important to be aware of your feelings about each treatment option when you are making your choices.

Hypnosis, imagery, and meditation, as well as herbs and supplements, all have their benefits and can adversely affect the cancer. Your doctor might say, "I don't know about them so don't take them." But that should not prevent you from doing your own research and finding some alternative treatments that might work well for you.

Christine talks about no longer identifying with her cancer. Yes, that is vital so that you are not living a role as a cancer survivor. Continue to create your authentic life and not focus on and empower your disease. She says, "I am grateful to be alive"; and it is very important for you to find things to be grateful for if you are to survive. Once you are grateful, the nightmares cease to exist. They have been confronted and reduced to a size that is easy to handle and overcome. Then your body knows you love life and it supports your effort to survive.

Happiness is about making the choice to be happy. That message cannot be repeated too often. You will find happiness by listening to the wise one who dwells within you.

My Tree of Life

Marie Mead

I don't remember that it was a particularly cold day, but I recall feeling chilled to my bones. I stood in the parking lot, shivering, trembling. Just minutes earlier, I had sat facing the oncologist, discussing a complete hysterectomy and removal of lymph nodes in my groin and lower back as calmly as if I had been talking to my hairstylist about taking off a couple of inches.

While talking with the cancer specialist, the surgery had sounded so routine. But then the enormity of it hit me as I stood in the parking lot; I finally weaved my way to the car on clumsy legs. I don't remember anything else about that day or the ones that immediately followed. A kind of numbness enveloped me and my mind was foggy.

I was relieved when my more proactive nature surfaced, and I started doing positive things for myself. Reading was an important step. Passages in *Love, Medicine, and Miracles* spoke to my soul and gave me courage. I also reviewed the biopsy results, consulted with others about options, and found a doctor who agreed to a less aggressive medical approach. He consented to treat me only after I promised to undergo frequent testing and to have major surgery if he was dissatisfied with my improvement. The delay in surgery gave me time to research traditional and alternative modalities of treatment. Working with the doctor, I combined treatments that seemed appropriate for me, made some lifestyle changes, and ultimately recovered.

That was eighteen years ago. The threat of a cancer recurrence or of other major illness didn't often come to mind. Until three weeks ago.

Feeling almost constantly fatigued was my first indication of something wrong. A sound sleep evaded me most nights. My concentration was affected. Food didn't agree with me, and I had pain of indeterminate origin. My eyesight seemed to abruptly deteriorate. I felt lousy, but I couldn't figure out why.

Still, I wasn't really concerned until I heard a different note in my doctor's voice. That's when I knew. He mentioned that my cancer markers were higher than they'd been in years, and I began to share his unease. He said more, but that is what I remember most clearly.

I was stunned, disappointed, scared. I was also angry with myself for some choices I'd made. Actually, one in particular. I had contracted to work on a project that turned out to be extremely stressful due to professional and ethical differences. Compounded with that were the loss of a loved one and a move across country. Wrapped up in the problems surrounding the project and my major life events, I lost track of what was truly important to me.

I examined my thoughts and realized that they often gave harsh commentary on my life. Instead of love and joy filling my days, I regularly felt anxious and disturbed. Negativity was my frequent companion.

Discussions with a psychotherapist gave me some much-needed perspective about the natural urges toward life—and about the myriad things that diminish vitality. What was my unconscious telling me? Was I being honest with myself about whether I would comfortably handle all that was happening in my life? Or was I sometimes feeling resentful and giving in to a sense of hopelessness? It didn't take much reflection to come up with the answer.

At various times in my life, I have tried to analyze and address any unfinished business that might get in the way of living life fully. I recognized that both the threat of cancer and the frustrating work with my project partner belonged under the "life-depleting" column. In contrast, the "life-affirming" column listed things that brought me joy but, sadly, were not occurring often enough in my life. Given the state of my health, it was readily apparent that I needed to strengthen my joy and my will to live.

It had been a while since I had seriously undertaken personal study, but now it was time to address my doubt and fear. I had been carrying them around in a private backpack, as though they were worthy of being treasured. I figured if I gave up carrying all that "stuff," my body would have more energy for healing.

I decided to heed my therapist's advice and listen to what the small inner voice was saying about my heart's desire. I needed some time to reflect and reestablish my perspective. Handing over the responsibilities for my precious, life-giving companion animals to pet-sitters, I drove to western North Carolina. Seeing the area for the first time, I was taken in by the beauty. It spoke to me, calling me to feel it to my core. I found a remote place to hike, and headed into the woods.

Some trees were toppled over, perhaps by the wind, and I recalled how I'd been laid low during the storms in my life. I climbed higher and higher. At regular intervals, I had to stop to catch my breath. My heart was pumping hard; my leg muscles were strained. I began laughing and once I started, I couldn't stop.

"You fool," I said between gasps for breath, "you don't have to worry about cancer. As out of shape as you are, you'll have a heart attack first!"

The humor of the situation took all the anxiety and fear right out of me. At the edge of a meadow, I watched a whirling vortex pick up the autumn leaves, sending them high into the air. It was a kaleidoscope of shapes and color, spinning and dancing in the sunlight—a visual delight!

Answers slowly unwound from that spiral of energy. I was starting the autumn of my life but, unlike the falling leaves that transform into humus and lend themselves to renewal, I was stuck and holding on to thoughts that were dragging me down.

I began listening, really listening, to the birds adding their song to the autumn color and beauty. The leaves falling from the towering trees were every hue of purple, red, green, yellow, and orange. Two butterflies, neon yellow in the sunlight, danced above me in the breeze. A bush covered with delicate white flowers gave nectar to more of the winged beauties. I realized that all around me were signs of transformation, and that I needed—and wanted—to be a part of it.

I stretched out my arms, hands open. Closing my eyes, I began to pray. Some leaves flitted through my fingers. As they did, I consciously let go of any thoughts about the hurtful actions of others; I also forgave myself. The negative thoughts fell to the ground with the leaves. Enfolding the process in prayer, I gave them over to God, the one Source.

Silence enveloped me. I have no idea how long I stood there, but all of a sudden I became conscious that my feet had grown roots into the soil. I was becoming like the trees, nourished by all that the earth gives forth. I was surprised by the depth of my roots, spreading deep into the earth, giving me life. Courage flowed upward, filling my being. As I reached toward the sky, my branches spread wide, my heart overflowed with love as birds sang from my extended arms. When they took wing, my heart soared with them on the wind, filled with hope.

Leaves began to rain down on me. Each carried its mystery of life, its secret message of joy, love, and peace.

And at that moment, I found my peace. I recognized that the present is a gift, each moment a treasure, perfect and right. I had been brought to this place due to concerns about my health and my negative choices. I was leaving renewed.

As I headed out of the forest, I felt lighter and filled with resolve. Everything was intensely perfect. The blue of the sky was clear and pure, decorated by wisps of white and an occasional soaring bird. It felt glorious. It *was* glorious!

Too soon, it was time to head back. I'd occasionally stop on my return down the trail, savoring each instant in this place.

As I perched on a rock, a tiny jumping spider inserted himself into my awareness time and again, until I realized that my large presence was between him and his mate. I took the couple as a good omen.

The pathway to the car was covered with moving leaves, running and skipping across the ground. It looked as though they were playing, celebrating their freedom after months of being bound to the trees. I'd never thought of the falling leaves in that way before—but what a joyful way to think of my autumn years: a time of play, celebrating my freedom from the sometimes arduous journey through adulthood.

"*Yes!*" I heard myself whisper aloud.

I drove straight to the hotel, wanting to relish my time alone. I retrieved from my suitcase *365 Prescriptions for the Soul*, brought along for inspiration. The beautiful cover had a tree on it. I smiled at the synchronicity of trees as the motif of the day.

The book opened to an often-read passage, Prescription 241.

If we are busily performing deeds but never stop to reach up for knowledge and wisdom, our tree of life will have no branches and many roots. Without branches, how can it move and respond with the winds of life? Or if we accumulate great knowledge but perform no deeds, then we are like a tree with many branches but no roots, and we will be blown over by the winds of fortune.

We must see that our tree of life contains both wisdom and deeds. Then our branches will spread and our deep roots will provide support and nourishment. We will be able to survive the storms and droughts that life presents us.

What a wonderful confirmation of my experience. Joyful tears filled my eyes and I offered a prayer of gratitude. I made a commitment to changing my life, holding fast to my dreams, and immersing myself in beauty and in the healing power of love.

I made another promise to myself: to be a willing collaborator with the great Author of my life, the one true Source. All I had to do was remember that I am a spiritual being having a human experience. It sounded so easy, but I knew from past experience that I often forget that truth. But I also knew that no matter which way I turned, to the right or left, God would be with me.

I now live on the edge of illness and I don't know what the future holds, but that's all right. I awaken to this beautiful place and feel immense joy fill my heart. I'm very lucky to have received a wake-up call, a reminder to live my dreams and to take some lessons from the trees.

BERNIE'S REFLECTION

As a tree can grow around nails, you, too, can take in
what irritates you and go on with your life.

This is a beautiful story showing you how to refocus your life and make the transition from death to life. Marie's first reaction was one of denial—everything sounded routine. That's still better than feeling hopeless as it relates to surviving. Then, what she calls her proactive spirit moved in. Once she had developed a fighting spirit, her chance for survival improved. This type of fight isn't focused on the cancer, but on what you can do to help yourself be a survivor by fighting for and reclaiming your life.

Marie immediately realized what was important in her life when she was faced with the possibility of being here only for a limited time. We all must learn, and remember, to say no when our heart says it does not feel right doing what has been asked of us. Your proactive spirit needs to know that you can and will start to say yes to yourself and your desires and needs. When you heal your life, you are far more likely to cure your disease as a side effect.

Marie had the courage to seek coaching on this path, to see a therapist, and to ask questions about herself so that she could learn what needed to be done to reclaim her life. You don't have to drag the backpack filled with the wounds of your past for your entire life. You can let go and abandon the parts of your past that are hurting you and remember you are a divine child.

One of the most important messages Marie shares is the value of humor and laughter. When you are laughing, you cannot be afraid. Fear cannot exist in the presence of joy and laughter. Studies show that cancer patients with a sense of humor live longer. So let your playful inner child come out and enjoy the moment.

I always talk about the fall leaves in my lectures, and finish with a slide of radiant autumn trees, representing this spiritual and meaningful time. I explain that if we live our lives as green leaves on the family tree in order to please everyone else, we lose our lives because we never really live for our own desires. When you realize the fall of your life has arrived, you shed the green and show your own uniqueness and beauty through an array of brilliant colors.

We often take the little things in nature for granted. For Marie, the tiny spider became something to admire as she saw it with new eyes. I encourage you every morning, before you leave home, to try to see everything as if you had never seen it before or are visiting this planet for the first time. Then when you step outside, you will truly see how many things there are to admire and how beautiful life is, from the leaves crackling under your feet and flowers blooming in the sun, to the many creatures, types of weather, and more. All of nature will become beautiful; just as the little spider was to Marie.

The Visitor

Randall Pease

Just as when the effluent-rich Sacramento River near my house clouds the Sierra-fed American River at the confluence, so, too, has an undercurrent of cancer merged with my native river of poetry to create a broader river on its way to the Delta and the sea. I am at home recovering from surgery for esophageal-gastric cancer at home. If you are walking or running around the park, you may see me mincing along. I am not casing the area; I am surviving, and grateful for this.

Haunted by an escalating set of symptoms—I had such difficulty swallowing at an annual Christmas party, I could not even finish a beer—I finally forced my way past my primary care doctor to a specialist. The gastroenterologist ordered an endoscopy to uncover the boulder that had interrupted the flow of my digestive system. I was sure it was an ulcer, caused by teacher overload. But before the endoscopy revealed the cancer, I had an unexpected visitor in my life: a vision.

I was teaching my twelfth-graders a poem about redemption. We examined and explored it by translating it into pictures. Finally, inspired by its message of hope, we began to write our own lyric in class. As my first-period students struggled to begin their poems, I modeled the composition process by writing my own poem in front of them. That was when a poetic visitor knocked on the door of my consciousness.

The Visitor

When night falls
like the limp hand,
almost translucent,
of my mother
on the hospital bed sheets,
another she,
a waif, slight, bedraggled,
in wispy, milk-white dress,
winds her weary way
from door to door.
No one lets her in,
her knocking is so light;
but I do.
And when I open my home
to her subtle entreaty,
she stares
from outside this world
like some deer caught in the headlights,
frozen still, ashamed, transparent,
but smiling.

With a hiss, slowly
she dissolves to mist, and slips in a whispering stream,
with a grateful sigh,
through the screen door.
She dampens my sweater
as she weeps through
and slides with her knife
of air
beneath my skin.
She blooms there.

She loves darkness;
like mushrooms
she grows inside,
and embraces me
and I her.
She is mine.

This homeless spirit who visited the house of my body remained nameless. It took me five periods of English to record the full story of this visitation. After school, the doctor explored my insides with his scope. In second period the next day, my wife called with the news to confirm the fate my prophetess had hinted at: the tumor was cancerous.

I was stunned. Addicted to exercise, I had none of the risk factors associated with cancers. Friends and family clenched their fists and advised me, "Fight it!" or "Beat it!" I demurred on that strategy. This was no fight. It was a visitation. This cancerous tumor was a part of me; I did not want to create an enemy within myself, with hostility on either side, thus hardening both positions. Those clenched fists, furrowed brows, and stiffened stomach muscles would turn my body into its own enemy.

That poetic visitor taught me how to approach my cancer. For no apparent reason, I was unlucky. The proper way to greet this Lady Luck, perhaps the homeless waif in my poem, was not to slam the door in her face, and certainly not to engage her in battle, but to welcome her, and then politely invite her to move on. The anger that cancer victims sometimes feel must be directed at someone or something, and I knew from my literary discipline that all such transcendent targets are merely metaphors; to me, there was no one to blame.

Cancer, however, does brand its victim, as if it were Hester Prynne's scarlet letter. The temptation is to consider cancer a judgment, either righteous, as a punishment for some transgression, or unfair, as an unprovoked attack that leads to self-pity and cynicism. I would rather not attribute morality where there is none. Cancer is simply a visitor, and I welcomed her with equanimity; in this way, I set myself free.

Because I refuse to read malignancy into the face of this visitor, she no longer has power over me. Because I am not focused on myself as a victim, coloring the world around me with the furrowed brows, the shadows of bad intentions, I am free to see the world clearly, and appreciate the birds, the sun, my family, and all the friends who have stood by me.

On the morning of my last day in the hospital, I shuffled around the fourth floor with my surgeon. We discussed my new body, what a lymph node is—a bean-shaped organ that helps deliver messages, and cancer, from node to node around the body—and the implications of chemotherapy. After our talk, I convinced my nurse I could venture downstairs on my own to buy the morning paper.

I meandered down what felt like subterranean hallways and up and down stairs. I did not know where I was, but finally saw an explosion of color and light, the outside with its flaming green trees and blazing blue sky. I bought my paper at the coin-operated newspaper box, then stopped. The sunshine, the red and yellow flowers, even the sounds of construction poured into me like a shower of gold. With a sigh of gratitude, I leaned against a column near the hospital entrance. A new person was being born in that moment. In the ashen, fluorescent depths of the hospital, this new persona had sprouted like a mushroom, secretly. Now, resurrected in the open air, I bloomed, a daffodil, out of that blind bulb that had been buried within the hospital.

I closed my eyes and soaked in the sun. Finally I turned to face the hospital, and, shocked, recognized where I was.

Nine days earlier I had entered those same doors on the way into surgery. Elated, I stepped into the waiting room, and reintroduced myself to the volunteer who had admitted me before. I had completed my redemptive circle. As I climbed the four flights of stairs to return to my floor, each stair was a step into another world. Apparently, when I answered the door to "The Visitor" that day in class, I had not just welcomed in someone new, cancer, but I had also released someone new, the newborn I had become, a cancer survivor.

BERNIE'S REFLECTION

Invite your monsters in, for you have much to learn
from them.

To me the river Randall describes relates to our bloodstream and how it can course through life and manage to overcome the

obstacles and redirections that life inevitably places before us.
It is only when we cease to flow and put up a dam that we stop
our progress and turn our life from a river into a trickling stream
devoid of energy, power, and direction.

His poem about the visitor is no accident. We are well aware
of our future at an unconscious level, and so art and poetry
often reveal the unknown to make it conscious and help us to
heal. I love the detail that it awakens him to the fact that there
is no enemy within him and nothing to fight. His energy isn't
misdirected into a battle and he does not feel any guilt. Thus he
can proceed to heal himself and his life.

When a monster appears in your dream, don't run away,
but do as Randall did and invite it in. He invites his visitor in
and welcomes her. The next thing we all need to do without
any guilt and blame is to ask our own visitor, "Why are you here
now? What may I learn from you about myself, my life, and
the changes that need to occur?" Randall is a teacher, and his
monster can be a teacher. Then, as the monster shares, it has no
power over you. It actually becomes a gift, as any teacher is who
helps you to grow.

Randall talks about his redemption, and he shares the fact that
he will be born again just as a seed or bulb creates new life. We
are all daffodils, able to grow, bloom, and blossom. I am always
amazed at the wisdom and determination in seeds. Think of the
role model a seed represents. It knows which way to go to find
the sun even when it is buried beneath the surface. It doesn't ask
what the odds are of being able to break through the pavement
and find the light of day. It just keeps growing until it finds its
way to be redeemed and bloom. To all of you I say, be that seed!
Do not let the growth gone wrong take over your life. Be the
growth and let your life blossom.

Standing Up for My Body and Soul

Andrea Hurst

I couldn't believe it, a second notice from my PPO plan in the mail notifying me that I was at high risk for breast cancer and should get a mammogram. What the heck were they bothering me for?

I'm just over forty years old, live a healthy lifestyle, and do not even own a microwave. There is no history of breast cancer in my family. I had thrown the first notice away and was tempted to do the same thing with this one, but a nagging voice crept in my head and said at least get a baseline for the future. Over the years I have learned to listen to my intuition, but I really did not want to take the time and go through the hassle of making the appointment. Two notices—well, perhaps there might be a message here for me.

Reluctantly I went for the mammogram. I promptly forgot about it until my phone rang at work and a faraway voice proceeded to tell me, "There is an area on the pictures that we have some concern about, we would like you to come in and see a surgeon soon."

Everything seemed to stop in the moment. I just stared out the window of my office at the tall pines. A *surgeon*, wasn't that an overreaction? Surgeons are for cutting; surely this was a mistake, and I did not have cancer. My mind slipped back to my father; is this what he had thought before his diagnosis? This was February and I had just sat by his bedside last November and watched him die from advanced prostate cancer. The grief still clung to my heart, and the thought of having cancer myself was just too much to bear.

I entered the surgeon's office, heart pounding, feeling like this was a bad dream, then put on a gown and covered my shivering body with my sweater. The door opened and a young, good-looking man walked in with copies of my mammogram film and put them up on a light box. He was the doctor, and he pointed to an area and in a very matter-of-fact way told me he would do a lumpectomy and it was scheduled for two weeks. My mind registered: there would be no biopsy first, they must be very concerned.

Two weeks of waiting and wondering. All I seemed to be able to do was alternate one minute from panic and a full scenario of leaving my husband and young children behind, to thinking the doctors had to be wrong and this was a benign tumor. I couldn't take this overwhelming anxiety another minute, so I walked out the door for a walk in the nearby woods. As I relaxed and listened inside, once again my intuition whispered to me that this was what they thought it was.

On the day of the surgery I somehow checked into the hospital and did deep breathing until they brought me in. The next thing I knew, I was awake and the room was spinning, the nausea overwhelming. In the haze I saw my surgeon with a somewhat smug smile on his face. I knew immediately, without a word from him, that it was cancer and that he was pleased with himself for making the call correctly. I could hear his words, but they were not registering: "It is an aggressive type of cancer, but still small enough to be categorized at this point as stage I. I suggest another surgery to remove lymph nodes, and a bone scan to see if the cancer has spread." A kind nurse came in and took one look at me and asked me if I understood. I just stared at her: how could I ever understand something like this happening to me?

Everything is moving very quickly now. Each diagnosis is a new piece of this puzzle I have to unravel—bone scan clean, no spreading into lymph nodes, suggest chemotherapy, suggest radiation, listen to us, listen to us. I have to make these decisions about my body and my life, ultimately for and by myself. I feel lost and unheard in this medical system of running everyone with the same diagnosis through the same treatment options like a well-oiled machine. I look on my bedside table at the book my friend gave me, *Love, Medicine, and Miracles*. I could use all of that about now, I think as I reach for the book and open it up.

As I turn the pages, for the first time since the diagnosis, I don't feel alone. I am laughing at Dr. Siegel's comments, crying at the parts that touch me, and feeling strong within myself. This book reminds me that I do not need permission from someone else to listen to myself and follow my own inner guidance to make choices about the best healing method for my body and soul.

I embark on an exhaustive search of treatment options, from traditional medical to alternative, natural, and spiritual. I read every type of research and make appointments with three cancer specialists, a naturopathic doctor, a chemotherapist, and a radiation physician. Each piece of data, each opinion I weigh against my overly sensitive body type and emotional and spiritual beliefs. What will work for *me*, not just any body, but *my* body?

In quiet contemplation, I pray to release the fear within me from all the dark images and possible case scenarios the doctors have told me could happen if I don't do it their way. I ask that love guide me, and visualize living to see my children grow up. I ask for healing and clear direction for the choice of treatments. Then I call my family together and tell them, "I have decided to do chemotherapy, no radiation, all in conjunction with various natural/alternative therapies and spiritual healing." I look around at their faces; some look relieved, others look afraid. I would like to please everyone, but know now that I must put myself first.

The music is blasting from the stereo as I choose my various options for my "Chemo Tape." I include Bernie Siegel's humor and jokes, peaceful classical music, and empowering songs. I play this tape on the way to the first chemo appointment and through the treatment. Now my mother is taking me to her house to rest and see how I will respond. The next thing I know, I am so nauseous, sick, and anxious that all I can do is pace. I try drugs to treat the side effects and only feel worse as the day goes on. There is no way I will be able to handle this chemo with my body, I know this at a very deep level. I also know that the cancer is gone from my body and that these chemo drugs will be damaging and are not necessary. Now how do I tell my doctors, family, and friends?

Curled under a blanket, I begin again to pray for guidance and direction and the strength to listen and follow up on how I am directed. I remember my mother telling me that as a baby I almost died from allergic eczema and none of the doctor's remedies worked. She took me to a Christian Science practitioner, who did a treatment on me. The practitioner then told my mother to give me back regular food again and let go of her fear and I would be well . . . and I was. For me, God as I know the Divine Power is the ultimate healer, and that is how I would be healed this time again.

Ultimately I decide no more chemotherapy. I tell my decision to my disappointed and highly distressed doctors and family with a calm determination, and proceed to put my own treatment agenda together. As part of that, I allow myself to play and feel joy in each day, to meditate and walk, to choose healthy foods and herbs, and to work with a set of natural and spiritual health practitioners. Each day feels like a blessing. I know I am taking a risk, but I also remember in Bernie's book that survivors stand up for themselves and sometimes really rock the boat! The most amazing side effect of my cancer is that it has brought me back to life and to a better understanding and love for myself. With consistent monitoring with medical doctors and standard tests, it has been over fifteen years that I have remained in complete remission.

BERNIE'S REFLECTION

Don't be afraid to ask the tough questions.

You must be an active participant in your treatment and evaluate what works and feels best for you. Doctors can tell you how a treatment works and its potential benefits and consequences, but what they cannot tell you is exactly how that treatment will affect your body. So doing everything doctors and health practitioners prescribe without listening to your own inner voice may not be your best survival behavior. You want to be an active participant, not a submissive sufferer. If your choices are based totally on your fears, then you tend to do everything everyone else prescribes so you won't feel guilty about making your own choices. But if your decisions are also about what you feel is right for you, then there are times you will say no to your doctor and family. Always listen to your body's inner wisdom, as Andrea did. When she realized that chemotherapy was not right for her, she explored other treatments and found ways to empower herself through her decisions. Her own method of treatment brought her back to herself and provided a better understanding of what it means to be alive. If she had done what didn't feel right, then she would have suffered far more side effects due to her inner conflict.

The personality of survivors propels them toward action, wisdom, and devotion. In other words, they take an active role in meeting their needs. They search for information to help them make decisions, and do not simply rely on the words and prescriptions of others. So don't be afraid to ask questions and do research about alternate treatment options. Make sure the doctor explains the reasons a certain treatment would be beneficial or how it could be harmful. When you give yourself permission to be involved in your treatment, you reclaim your life.

Many of us have given up our lives to please others or are going through treatment simply because others want us to. But they are not going through the treatment. As I have said, the issue is, am I choosing what is right for me? As I have said before, for me death is not a failure, but not living is. Knowing what is right comes from heart wisdom, not head wisdom. To help determine which treatment is right for you, you may try drawing images of the various options. Patients who are contemplating chemotherapy, and then go on to draw the treatment as beautiful golden light eliminating their cancer, are receiving a positive sign from their inner wisdom to help them make their choice.

The key is in not just getting information, but in combining it with inspiration. You have to have a will to live, self-esteem, and self-love to help you survive. Learn to love yourself and trust your judgment. Take control of your health and take control of your life. As one young woman wrote to me, "Cancer made me take a look at myself and I like who I met." Yes, there are many side effects to cancer and its treatment, and some are truly wonderful.

Write It Down, Pass It On

Carol Westfahl

It was a grocery store trip not unlike the thousands of other trips I've made in my adult life. I wandered up and down the aisles pushing the squeaky wire cart, pausing to consider one loaf of bread over another, trying to remember which brand of toothpaste I'd been buying lately or whether it was time to restock on Kleenex. Finally I arrived at the one section I'd been avoiding—school supplies.

School supplies, doesn't that sound harmless? Pens, pencils, blank paper, and crayons all bought in happy anticipation by children with their lives ahead of them. Well, I wasn't there for a box of crayons. What I needed was a notebook, a blank notebook I could fill with information. Information about lymphoma, the cancer I'd just been told I had.

I scanned the small selection of spiral-bound notebooks, my eye settling on purple. My favorite color, purple. Purples and mauves and burgundies, colors I used in my house to create the mood I liked. Maybe a purple notebook could carry me through the coming ordeal, I thought, as I tossed it into the squeaking cart and steered toward the checkout counter.

I used that purple notebook every day. Sitting down at day's end, I made careful note of doctor's appointments, diagnoses, treatment options, prescriptions, specialists, and results. This was not a flowery account of my cancer journey, it was a plain, white-bread, and generic account of what was going on. It made me feel I had the situation under control, that it was just another work-related assignment like the many I'd completed in my decades on the job with the State of Wisconsin. And soon enough, the treatment was over, the cancer was gone, and I was headed back to my office after months of working from home. I packed everything having to do with lymphoma in a "cancer box," tossed in that purple notebook, sealed up the box with packing tape, and put it in the back of the garage. The end, at last.

Ah, but my story doesn't end there, does it? With me in my office and everything else back in place. For a few years after the cancer left, it was like that: a tidy daily routine of dressing for work, the commute on icy Wisconsin roads, the office filled with familiar coworkers, the day filled with projects large and small, all needing completion.

No, my cancer story goes on, because six years later the lymphoma returned. Six years had passed, some 1,800 more days at the office. This time, when the doctor gave me the news, I thought, "Enough." I thought I'd paid my dues the first time, but no. Here it is again. I'm going to do it differently this time. Right then and there I decided to quit my job.

A job I'd loved for years, but it was time to retire and devote myself to a different kind of living. A life, a daily life, in which I'd do whatever I wanted. The time had come for me to take care of my own needs instead of routinely fulfilling others' expectations. My coworkers were stunned by my abrupt announcement. I spread the word that I wanted no retirement party or fuss made over my leaving, but a few gifts showed up anyway. I held one small package in my hand and knew right away what it was under the wrapping. "A journal," I thought as I felt the outlines with my fingers. "Good, I'll be needing another one of these."

And I did. Instead of digging out that faded purple spiral notebook filled with dry facts and information, I sat down and opened up that pretty little journal and picked up my pen to let my emotions pour out on the page. Page after page—all in ink pen, mind you, there was no going back once I put my thoughts and feelings down on the blue-lined paper. Yes, once again I sat in my cozy den at night and wrote about doctor's visits and treatments, but this time I added what was really happening, that before office visits I was on my knees praying. That I was in pain. That I was angry. My emotions were suddenly close to the surface, and I decided to let them stay there.

My emotions were still close to the surface the day my doctor told me the words we all long to hear—that my lymphoma was now in remission. I left the office with tears in my eyes and walked out into the parking lot. On impulse I walked past my parked Honda, always reliable in the Wisconsin cold. I kept walking across the entire lot, and across four lanes of commuter traffic to a nature trail I could see in the distance along Lake Michigan. I needed to be surrounded by nature while I absorbed this new information. I was no longer afraid, I was no longer angry. I was relieved, I was grateful. But in many ways, I was also confused. Hunched against the cold in my thin coat and street shoes, I walked along the frozen shoreline, my surging emotions keeping me warm.

I thought back to a moment early in my first struggle with cancer. I'd been reading *Love, Medicine, and Miracles* and came across Bernie Siegel's question: what are the benefits to having this disease? I was angry when I read that passage. In fact, the very idea that he could ask it made me livid, I wanted to toss his book into the fireplace and just burn it up. Now, years later, I could see that maybe he was right, and my benefit had finally arrived. As I walked I looked up to the sky, and suddenly it occurred to me that I had a few questions for God.

"What am I supposed to do with this time I've been given, God? What is the plan?" A new life was stretching ahead of me, curving like the bends along the shore. A life without doctors, treatments, and, best of all, without a cancer journal.

I was now in the habit of writing, though. Not only had my evening writing served as a release for my emotions, but I'd also come to take growing delight in words and communicating. I liked putting my thoughts on paper. I liked writing in ink, watching the words piling up behind my pen. "God, could I keep on writing?" I asked again. "I don't want to leave that part of my old life behind."

By the time I returned to my parked car that afternoon so many years ago, I did have a plan, one that God helped me see on my walk along the lake. I could take what I'd learned on my two cancer journeys and use that information to help others. I could put my pen to paper and pass the knowledge from one survivor to another in an endless chain of encouragement and understanding. I didn't have to seal up my words in a box and put them on the garage shelf; instead I could send them out into the world as my way of helping others. Cancer gave that to me, and for that I am grateful.

BERNIE'S REFLECTION

When you listen to your inner self, your decisions become easier to make.

There are many aspects of survivor wisdom in Carol's evolving changes and activities. The value of a journal in which you can express feelings is critical and very therapeutic. Journaling allows you to listen to yourself and hear your true inner voice. During difficult times, it can sometimes be inspiring to reread your own words again. By keeping your innermost thoughts and deepest secrets within the pages of a notebook, you can look back and see the roller coaster of emotions that go with your life experiences. You can laugh, cry, or even be embarrassed by yourself, but you always come to a better understanding of who you are. Journaling is a great way of keeping track of your personal and spiritual development. Carol's favorite color, purple, symbolizes the resources represented by her spiritual side. I often use drawings to see what colors people draw themselves in, and what colors they use to depict their disease and treatment. These drawings reveal unconscious meanings, which can affect treatments and their outcome. Through the new awareness of her feelings that she gained from her journal, Carol walked away from the demands of her job and transformed her life. She learned how to stop thinking and start feeling what was right for her and her life.

Carol's anger at me and my philosophy was a good sign because it led to action rather than sinking into depression and guilt. I am never upset when people get angry at what I have written, because the anger is energy. If they curl up in bed feeling guilt, shame, and blame because of what I wrote, we both have a problem. For those who have gone through cancer, keeping a journal of emotions is a way of expressing the anger, fear, and frustration that come with the diagnosis. Simply by acknowledging these feelings, you have already begun to heal. With her second journal, Carol decided to face her emotions and keep them on the surface.

It is very easy for someone experiencing a myriad of feelings to want to turn off all emotion and focus on the cold statistics and facts of their condition, as Carol did with her first journal. Most people try to become numb or distracted, but that is not survival behavior. Though it is important to keep track of the physical aspects of the disease, when you ignore your emotional components and feelings, you can miss the opportunity to connect with others in a similar situation. Carol's journal helped her discover her passion for writing and increased her desire to share her experience with others who may be in need of an expressive outlet for their feelings. Just as Carol found inspiration in her own words, she then used her writing to give hope to others.

Thumz Up

Joe Underwood

Does it get any better than this?" I asked myself when I learned I'd been chosen from the thousands of teachers nationwide as a Disney Teacher Award Honoree. Me? Amazing! I couldn't wait to join the other teachers, a class of thirty-nine honorees assembled at Disneyland in California in July for an amazing week of parties, parades, and a gala befitting rock stars and actors. What a thrill! I couldn't believe I'd been included in this bunch. After our week together in Anaheim, we were all to get together again a few months later in Orlando, Florida. A lot can change in just a few months, though, can't it?

Everyone was anxiously looking forward to our Orlando gathering, and e-mails of anticipation were becoming more and more exciting. My plans were in place, I had convinced my principal that this opportunity would be very worthwhile, and I was even able to convince some administrators in my school district to cover substitute pay in my absence. How important was this trip? I even rearranged my football officiating schedule since I would be missing some game assignments. How dare they plan a professional development education conference during football season! Everything was right and ready to go.

And then I got sick. I didn't get sick, actually, since I officiated five football games that week, but I did wake up one Sunday morning suffering from stomach cramps. I dismissed this discomfort, but my wife, Nancy, who handles these types of situations much better than I, insisted on taking me to the emergency room. So, off we went. Seventeen hours and three CT scans later, I found myself on a gurney being wheeled from ER to OR for surgery. A lump had been discovered in my colon. It was removed.

Sounded good to me, now let me go home.

After a week of hospitalization I finally convinced my doctor, whom I kept referring to as "Dr. Discharge," to let me go home. I was positive that I was ready. It was Friday morning and Dr. Discharge eventually signed me out, but not before I had a meeting with an oncologist, Dr. Fu (I had no idea what an oncologist was up to this point). Dr. Fu, however, let me know pretty quickly what she was up to. She explained that I had cancer and told me I would have to undergo chemotherapy treatments. She also said I would have to make some compromises.

"I can't," I told her, "I have too many things to do."

"You will," she replied, "or you won't have to worry about what you have to do."

My life had now abruptly changed. Everything changed. I was going to be out of school for some time (totally unacceptable); I had to immediately give up officiating football, not for a week, but an entire season (a devastating loss); and my upcoming trip to be with my fellow Disney honorees was in jeopardy (only two weeks away).

My biggest concern still had to be addressed: what about my Disney meeting in Orlando? It was coming up in eight days. I had planned to drive and still intended to do so. Nancy was concerned that sitting and driving for four hours, alone, would be too much. I was positive that everything would be fine. Doctor Fu told me I could go if I felt well enough. I would still be recovering from surgery, and my chemo treatments were still a few weeks away. I decided I would probably go; actually, I knew I would go, but I told Nancy I would "probably" go. She knew that I would go, too, but she didn't let on. I e-mailed my fellow honorees and told them I was going to be in Orlando.

After a weekend of unrest, I returned to school on Tuesday. I met with my kids; their concern was genuine and really heartfelt. I met with my principal; he questioned whether the Disney trip was a good idea. I convinced him that I was going to proceed as planned. I was leaving Saturday.

That Thursday I had an appointment for a bone marrow test. If you have never had a bone marrow test, don't. Actually, it was tolerable. After a mild sedative, a needle was inserted into my hip, into my bone, and into my iliac crest, and a sample of tissue was withdrawn. Okay, not so bad. Wait, now we will switch and do it all over again. Dr. Fu punctured my other hip and proceeded to take another tissue sample. While my bone marrow was sent to a lab for testing, I was sent home to get some rest. I needed it for my long drive coming up in less than twenty-four hours.

Driving in Florida is relatively easy compared to other states. It is all flat and straight. But if you have recently had surgery on your stomach and needles poked through your bones, I can assure you it is not especially comfortable. I felt like I had been taken into an alley and beaten: stabbed in my gut and blackjacked on my back. Other than that, my drive was great.

Since first becoming a Disney Teacher Award Honoree, I had been looking for something to symbolize my accomplishment, but I could never find exactly what I wanted. When I arrived in Orlando and checked into Disney's Contemporary Hotel, however, I finally found what I was looking for. It was a pin, of which there are hundreds to choose from, but this one caught my eye. On a rectangular field of red, bordered by a gold edge, was a Mickey hand giving a "thumbs-up" sign. Perfect! What a great symbol. Not only did I find my Disney "hand," but I had found something that most people usually associate with a positive attitude: a thumbs-up. I am positive I am going to overcome this cancer thing, so I wanted others to be just as positive as me. Also, one of my fondest memories growing up is of my father giving me a thumbs-up whenever I did something that pleased him. He would look at me, put up his thumb, and say, "Way to go buddy." This pin summed it all up. I wore it every day during our professional development.

Our honoree reunion and learning experience was wonderfully enriching. We began by thinking of a student we believed in and writing that student's name down on a piece of paper and putting it away. As our meetings progressed over those few days, a couple of my colleagues would point to my thumbs-up pin and remark how cool they thought it was.

Although none of us looked forward to our professional (and personal) development ending, Saturday came sooner than anyone wanted. All thirty-nine principals from our schools were there, plus the Disney staff and others, about eighty people altogether.

As we stood outside our hotel in a large circle for our final encounter, we spoke about that student whose name we had written down on day one. Progressing around our circle of eighty participants, students' names were stated and our individual and collective belief in them all kept pouring forth. As our circle of belief neared its end, a wonderful Disney teacher stated whom she believed in, and then she announced that there was one more item to address before we closed. She began reading a statement that said, in effect, "Joe, we believe in you and are behind you in your fight against cancer. We know you will overcome this obstacle because of your positive attitude, and we love you." Hearing that statement, I was taken by surprise and very touched. But she was not done. Everyone was staring at me as she continued, "Honorees, please take out your pins and put them on." At this point, every honoree plus everyone else in attendance pulled out a thumbs-up pin.

My heart was in my throat and tears rolled down my cheeks. Over eighty people dedicated those thumbs-up pins to me as a symbol of my struggle. They also promised to wear those pins every day until I go into remission. I was so overcome with heartfelt emotion, it was hard to breathe. I could not believe that this diverse group of wonderful educators would make such a dedication to one person—to me. Every one of them then approached me and gave me a hug, and every one of them has continued to wear his or her thumbs-up pin ever since.

I am told that many people asked the honorees about those pins, and now there are several hundred people, including students, wearing a thumbs-up pin as a reminder that someone—whom they don't even know—can overcome a fight against cancer.

I have not yet overcome my battle with non-Hodgkin's lymphoma, but I have survived my bout with chemotherapy. I had lost all my hair when our Disney group gathered for our final meeting that May back in Anaheim. When I arrived, I was so touched that every single person was wearing their thumbs-up pin. I still wear it today. That pin, and the support of my Disney teachers, has helped me get to full remission. Nothing in my professional life has been more magical. Thumz up!

BERNIE'S REFLECTION

You're all winners.

Every once in a while we hear about an act of kindness so remarkable, we are moved to tears. From people making anonymous donations to those who cannot afford to pay their medical bills, to a group of students shaving their heads to match their classmate who is going through chemotherapy, we can see that there is goodness in the world. What is truly amazing about Joe's story is that his attitude and will to live affected so many others and led strangers to wear the thumbs-up pin in support of his cause. His decision to go on the trip showed his dedication and determination to live his life and not let cancer hold him back. As the quantum physicists say, desire and intention alter the physical world, causing things to occur that would not normally occur if they were not desired. I always add the word "determination" to that statement, because I think that is also an essential part of creating change. From my perspective, although I don't like to think of it as a battle, Joe has already won the battle with cancer because he did not let it take away his will to live.

Joe became an inspiration to his fellow Disney teachers, and in return, they offered him support and became an inspiration to him. A Disney thumbs-up pin was the perfect token to help keep Joe's attitude positive. He associated it with the memory of his father and accomplishment. Through this association, Joe believed he could and would win the battle against cancer, and he helped others to share that belief. Missing school and not being able to participate in the football season were disappointing, but Joe learned to live each day, and take life just one day at a time.

When you have goals, like getting to Orlando or seeing your child grow up, you are far more likely to make it than the person who goes home, climbs into bed, and makes no effort to create what their heart desires.

I knew a college football player at Colgate, my alma mater, who when confronting leukemia so impressed the team that they planned to give him an award at one of the games. Due to his low white count from chemotherapy, they couldn't do it out on the field as they had planned, so they held a limited gathering in the locker room at halftime. The team was losing rather badly to Army at that time. When Mark entered the locker room he said, "When I wasn't playing, I always thought I gave everything I had on every play. But now that I am not playing, I realize that I didn't. So don't leave anything in here. Leave it all out there on the field." The team went out and upset Army and won the game. The key, however, is not the final score but the effort. We all will die, but how many of us will have truly lived?

When you have people who care around you giving you the thumbs-up, you suffer less pain and fewer side effects from your treatment. So we all need a team made up of caring "thumbs-up-ers." Life is a marathon, and we are here to finish the race and give it our best shot. Then you can never be called a loser. And when you give it your best shot and the fans are there cheering you on, the results can be amazing and no accident. I always remember that lady standing on a street corner in New York as I jogged my way through the New York City Marathon course saying to everyone who passed, "You're all winners." Joe Underwood certainly is a winner!

CONCLUSION

Love, Medicine, and Miracles Today

When I was about seven years old, our family was on vacation in Cape Cod. While walking down the street in Provincetown, I turned to my parents and said, "I'm going to be a doctor when I grow up." I have no memory of that moment or my decision, but heard it often enough from my parents that it must be true.

As a teenager who was skilled in art, I didn't know that some artists sold their work and earned a living doing what they loved. The only commercial side of art I could see was being a decorator, and that was not for me. But since I had skilled hands, loved people, liked to fix things, and was fascinated by science and nature, becoming a surgeon seemed like the way to participate in all my interests. The painful part, and what I was unprepared for emotionally, led me to where I am today.

Here's why—when you attend medical school, the faculty do not help you to understand how to cope with loss and the emotional aspects of medicine. There are many medical students who become physicians because they are fascinated by the human body. The problem is that actual people come in the body. One aspect of being a surgeon is that you are directly involved in the medical process—truly hands-on—and not just writing prescriptions. What is painful about this profession is the fact that sometimes, your decisions or the complications of surgery lead to more problems for your patients. I was not prepared for the pain related to all the things I couldn't fix for my patients, and I could get no answers from my teachers as to why God would make a world where children developed cancer and died.

It is not only the patients who are in pain. Doctors suffer from posttraumatic stress disorder, too. For me, my M.D. stood for "My Disease." Here is a great example of that. I have a portrait I painted of myself, done in 1977, hanging in our living room. But who is the painting really of? You wouldn't know it's me because I am hidden behind a surgeon's cap, mask, and gown. Doctors bury their pain and never discuss it at medical meetings or conferences. We do not feel, we think. Often, when you ask a doctor how it feels to be a doctor, they answer, "I think what it's like . . ." *Think?* Have you noticed that many famous paintings show doctors with sick and dying patients sitting with chin in hand thinking and not actually touching the patient? When I ask medical students to draw themselves working as a doctor, the vast majority hand me drawings with no people in them, just equipment and books, or they are sitting behind a desk with their diploma on the wall. If they are touching anyone, it is with a stethoscope. Imagine if these things were discussed in medical school in a therapeutic way. That would have helped me, as well as all the medical students who came after me, to find healthier reasons to become physicians.

Thirty years ago (the same year I painted the portrait), I wrote the dean of my medical school thanking him for making me a fine surgeon but telling him he did not teach me how to emotionally care for my patients or myself. What did I hear in reply? Nothing. He never answered my letter. Over the years, I have watched as medicine has let technology become the focus so medical students get medical information but not a medical education. Recently I sent a copy of the letter to the present dean of the same school, saying it was nice to see things changing, feelings being shared and the progress that was occurring. What did I hear from him? Nothing; he never answered my letter, either.

Early in my career, a veterinarian became my patient, and I told him I was going to give up my practice and go to veterinary school because I couldn't take the pain of dealing with people. He saved me and awakened me when he answered, "Don't, because people bring the pets in." He helped me to begin to see the people I was caring for as people and not as problems or diseases, and my journey to healing began. With that, I was on my way to being a better person and a better physician.

From then on, I took matters into my own hands and began to attend workshops. Doctors Carl Simonton, Elisabeth Kubler-Ross, and Karl Menninger were some of my teachers, and they helped me to open my mind and alter my experience so traditional beliefs no longer limited me. I had never encountered many of the things they taught, but I had the courage to deal with my feelings and seek the help I needed to avoid becoming numb to what was happening to my patients. I learned how meditation and guided imagery could make me aware of my inner wisdom and mind/body communication. I was amazed when Elisabeth Kubler-Ross took one look at a simple drawing I did and told me about my life. I learned about the value of dreams in relationship to somatic and psychological information.

However, the biggest factor that redirected my life was one of my own patients with breast cancer, saying the words that started me on my path to a new life. We were both at the same conference because of our pain. She sat next to me, no desk separating us as it did when she came to my office, and said, "You're a nice guy and I feel better when I'm in the office with you, but I can't take you home with me. So I need to know how to live between office visits." Suddenly I didn't have to feel like a failure. I could help people to live instead of trying to cure every disease and keep them from dying.

When I returned to the office, I moved my desk against the wall so I was no longer separated from my patients. I carried crayons with me to the hospital and got patients to draw pictures, and I began a new journey into the lives of the people I cared for and about.

My patients became my teachers. When I was hurting I would say, "I need to hug you." I thought I was helping my patients, but I finally realized the first words were "I need"; and my patients were healing me because they knew I needed help. Many times when I was ready to give up surgery, they wouldn't let me.

I have also learned to accept the criticism of my patients. I believe it helps polish my mirror and make me a better doctor. All of the best doctors are criticized by their patients, nurses, and families. Why? Because they apologize, are willing to learn, and do not make excuses or blame their patients. Therefore, people know these doctors are willing to listen to the constructive criticism and be coached. Those who deny their imperfections, make excuses, and blame others do not get criticized, because people learn they are wasting their time talking to them. Doctors who have never been patients are tourists, not natives, in the land of the experience of disease.

I have operated upon my mother-in-law, sister, and children, and have learned from them. While I felt as capable as any surgeon in handling their problems, I wanted them cared for by someone who also loved them. When our son Keith had a tummy ache, I examined him and discovered he had an inguinal hernia. As a trained pediatric surgeon, I made plans to operate upon him as an outpatient and took him to the hospital so he would see all the rooms and meet all the people who would be involved in his care. I thought I was preparing him properly for the event. When he woke up in the recovery room, I was standing by his side. He looked up at me and said, "You forgot to tell me it was going to hurt." That touched my heart and made me a better doctor. As a tourist I was learning from the natives.

When Keith was seven years old, after an X-ray of his painful leg revealed what appeared to be a malignant bone tumor, I thought he only had a short time left to live. I was quite depressed, to say the least. He came to me the next day and said, "Dad, can I talk to you for a minute? You're handling this poorly." So I keep learning about living in the moment from our pets and children. Keith turned out to have a very rare benign tumor, but I learned a great deal from him the week before his surgery.

I also learned from my family that you can't separate yourself from your life. When my wife gave birth to five children in seven years, including twins, both she and I were exhausted and became ill. My week in the hospital made me a much better doctor because now I had *lived* the experience and was again one of the natives instead of just a tourist. Because of my experience and desire to help people live between office visits, I decided to send a letter to all our cancer patients offering them a longer, better life if they came to a weekly group meeting.

I sent out one hundred letters and then went into a panic state because I forgot to say this offer was only for our patients. I expected several hundred people to show up for the first meeting, thinking everyone would bring their friends and relatives with cancer. Well, it turns out that I was wrong. Fewer than a dozen women came to the first meeting. It was quite a wake-up call that helped me realize I didn't really know the people I was caring for.

What I began to see was that the people who came were, as my wife, Bobbie, called them, *exceptional*. They were willing to express their emotions, read books, draw pictures, and change without the fear of doing it wrong. So we became the Exceptional Cancer Patients, or ECaP. To make a long story short, I also saw that when you helped people to live and empowered them to heal their lives, they didn't die when they were supposed to.

ECaP began thirty years ago. Our first meetings took place in bank boardrooms, churches, and anywhere we could get free space. As we developed, we were able to obtain funding through my books and audio recording sales, rent an office, and develop a staff available to run groups and present workshops. Today ECaP has its offices in Meadville, Pennsylvania, and is run by Doctor Barry Bittman and his wife, Karen. Our goal is to help people confronting cancer and other illnesses to become empowered and live. We have the Web sites www.ecap-online.org and www .berniesiegelmd.com.

Today there are many organizations doing support work, raising funds for research and more for cancer patients and others. I wish I had been a better businessman so I could have done more over the years to help. Let me say that what I learned about mind/body interplay is not limited to cancer. We help people with multiple sclerosis, AIDS, autoimmune diseases, chronic fatigue, fibromyalgia, and more. As a surgeon, I cared for more people with cancer, and so it was natural for me to start working with them and help them to live between office visits.

Back when ECaP was starting, I was excited, thinking I had discovered something about survival that would help other patients. So I started to write articles and send them to medical journals. These were articles discussing how changes in a patient's life and emotional state, dreams, and drawings affected his health and ability to heal. The editors sent my articles back, saying, "Interesting but inappropriate for our journal." Imagine that—the idea that it is inappropriate to discuss a patient's ability to heal. How could that be? That is one of the problems with medical literature. It is closed-minded, like a plumbing journal not wanting any articles by electricians. However, if physicians focus only on their limited field, they are not caring for their patients in a holistic and integrative fashion. Optimistically, I sent my articles to appropriate journals, and they were again returned with a note saying, "It's appropriate for our journal but not interesting."

Here is what I began to realize: all the things I was discovering about the benefits of healing patients' lives and mind/body interaction were known by those who were involved in psychiatry, psychology, and Jungian therapy, but not general medicine. I visited Susan Bach, a Jungian therapist, in London and we discussed the somatic (the holistic relationship of the body and mind) aspects of my drawings and how Jung was fascinated by these kinds of drawings. Yet as doctors, we are not taught to ask our patients to draw pictures to learn about the conscious and unconscious aspects of their somatic and psychic components.

Elisabeth Kubler-Ross's work with the dying and drawings made me aware that consciousness was not local. By nonlocal I mean that consciousness exists as an entity separate from the mind and body. Consciousness dictates what the mind mediates and has a universal presence not affected by time or place. Through Kubler-Ross, I met therapist Gregg Furth and learned even more from his work with drawings. I still have not met a medical student who has been told that Jung interpreted a dream and made a correct physical diagnosis. Just like faith, hope, and joy, our mind, body, and spirit are an interactive unit, and they must be appreciated and treated as a unit. Only then can true healing occur.

What I learned and experienced, I kept sharing with patients and their families. They needed to hear it—this was not about people being immortal but about survival behavior and the qualities that exceptional patients have, and that to have the best chance of surviving, others needed to develop these qualities, too. These are common themes that you can read or hear about in the Bible, in addiction groups, and from kids with cancer, Marines, therapists, survivors of concentration camps, and more. They are about surviving difficult times, and it doesn't matter what the threat is, but it does matter how the person responds to it.

After starting ECaP and seeing the benefits of support and empowerment groups to individuals and their survival, I began to go out and speak about my experiences. Several people came up to me at various lectures saying, "Remember me?" These were patients who were supposed to have died, but were alive and well. They had stopped coming back to the office because all they had heard were negative comments about their chances of surviving. Not from me, I might add, but from other physicians. Meeting these survivors reinforced my beliefs and experience.

One evening, someone came up to me and asked, "Have you ever thought about writing a book?" Me? Write? I wasn't sure. . . . I am very visual; my lowest grade in four years of college was a C in Creative Writing. But that question started the ball rolling, and the people appeared who helped me to write and publish my experiences in *Love, Medicine, and Miracles* in 1986 and many more books since then. When the book first came out and caused a lot of controversy, I was invited to be on the Oprah Winfrey show, I thought to praise me. I was joined on the show by other doctors who took issue with what I'd said and believed in. Due to dear Oprah, the book became a number-one best-seller; and twenty years later and over two and a half million copies sold, it is still being read all over the world, helping people to survive. However, I still can't get my college to raise my writing grade to a B.

At the time, my views and opinions challenged the system, and I got on all the popular talk shows because of this. My words and ideas disturbed a lot of other doctors, who said this was all nonsense. When the writer Norman Cousins talked and wrote about his experience with illness and self-healing, doctors didn't feel threatened because that was just a story. I was trying to make it scientific, but I was criticized for my lack of research. No one had been willing to finance my research because they didn't believe in what I was saying. When a Yale student did research with our ECap or exceptional cancer patients, his professor didn't believe the favorable results and altered the control group to change the outcome.

Today, research has been done to verify what I believed and the benefits it offers to the patients. Even the benefits of playing music in the operating room have been noted. When I first brought a tape recorder into the OR and played music, I was called an explosion hazard. When I talked to anesthetized patients, I was considered crazy. When I spoke at conferences, I was yelled at. Years later, when the benefits were apparent, I was invited to speak before the same conferences that earlier had shouted me down. And many of my treatment modalities became hospital policy because my end results were more successful and no one was against success. The most helpful were the doctors who did research to prove I was wrong and came out with the opposite results. What I was doing was not expressing anything new, but giving what was known a new form of expression.

Many doctors would say to me, "I can't accept that," after I would share a case or some information with them. Not that they couldn't explain or understand it, but that they couldn't accept it. The problem was that their minds were closed. If we brought these subjects into medical schools, I believe the students would be open to a different experience when they started practice. Today at Memorial Sloan-Kettering Cancer Center in New York they have an integrative medical department run by psychologist Barrie Cassileth. She told me that the administration favored it more than the medical staff did. Sad comment, but typical of medicine today. I always say, I prefer to talk to astronomers and quantum physicists because they are comfortable with uncertainty and know the effects of desire and intention.

I recall the renowned Doctor Karl Menninger telling me that after my book *Love, Medicine, and Miracles* came out, he was going to write a book called *Twelve Hopeless Cases*, about twelve people who were considered hopeless by doctors and were alive and well today. He said, "But I don't have to. You have written it." I began to find many books with the same message, but again, psychotherapists, rather than medical doctors, had written them.

Thankfully, today is a different day in medicine, and studies have been done showing the health, survival, and recovery benefits of having music in the operating room, putting up outdoor nature scenes in the hospital room, talking positively to anesthetized patients, having a sense of humor, spirituality, imagery and visualization, pets, relationships, and more.

As I began to shift my mode of practice from treating diseases to caring for people, some interesting things happened that helped me follow my path through life in the direction I was meant to go. As I was invited to speak to many groups, I began to make out the year's on-call schedule for myself and my four partners to avoid any conflict. One day my partner Bill McCullough said to me, "Did you notice how you mark the schedule?" I told him I didn't know what he was talking about. He went on to explain that since I was doing so much work with drawings and colors, it was interesting that I colored the days I was practicing surgery in black while the days I was away teaching and lecturing were clean and white. By pointing that out, he really helped me make an important decision. Put yourself in my shoes and think about giving up a career you love. It was not easy for me to stop doing surgery and shift my entire life into caring for people through my words, focusing on lectures, workshops, support groups, and teaching. His remark about the calendar helped me to see the truth at a deeper, meaningful, and even unconscious level.

Another factor that helped me to shift the focus of my life was that my audiences were beginning to include more health care practitioners. I was no longer the problem, but now was a source of information and a resource for both the doctor and the patient.

Would I still like to be operating? Yes, but I can help more patients by talking to them, their doctors, and hundreds of medical students than I could if I spent the same amount of time doing surgery.

Now, years after I was a controversial figure and sought-after talk show guest, I am not a source of conflict and trouble. People now agree with me, and science verifies my ideas. In his book *The Biology of Belief*, Bruce Lipton says it all very well. He calls genes "blueprints," and says it is the chemistry of our internal environment that selects which gene is activated. Identical twins don't develop the same disease on the same day. And when one does and the other does not, you need to take a look at their life stories for the reason. A recent study reveals how loneliness affects the genes that regulate immune function and makes you vulnerable to cancer, and to autoimmune and viral diseases.

This is not about blame, but about understanding that you cannot separate your health from your life experience. Mind, body, and spirit are all parts of a unified organism—you. There are so many examples in our daily lives about people developing cancer, and other illnesses, at times of enormous stress, loss, and change in their lives. Psychologists define these as "life crisis units."

Though some see it as controversial, I believe it is important to focus on these life crisis units, asking yourself what happened in the last two years before your diagnosis. I also think patients should ask themselves, "How do I benefit from an illness?" I now ask my patients a list of questions that define an immune-competent personality. It was created by psychiatrist Dr. George Solomon in his research with AIDS patients. He found that the answers to these questions defined who would be a long-term survivor of AIDS. If you answer no to the first seven questions and yes to the last two, you need attention.

1. Do I have a sense of meaning in my work, daily activities, family, and relationships?

2. Am I able to express anger appropriately in defense of myself?

3. Am I able to ask friends and family for support when I am feeling lonely or troubled?

4. Am I able to ask friends or family for favors when I need them?

5. Am I able to say no to someone who asks for a favor if I can't or don't feel like doing it?

6. Do I engage in health-related behaviors based on my own self-defined needs instead of someone else's prescriptions or ideas?

7. Do I have enough play in my life?

8. Do I find myself depressed for long periods during which time I feel hopeless about ever changing the conditions that cause me to be depressed?

9. Am I dutifully filling a prescribed role in my life to the detriment of my own needs?

To Solomon's list I add questions to see if people are in touch with their feelings and can accept their beauty and divinity.

1. I am taking you out to eat; what would you like for dinner?

2. What would you hang up in the lobby of every public building with a sign over it that says, look at how beautiful and meaningful life is?

3. How would you introduce yourself to God?

What I am hoping to hear from a patient is:

1. A quick response to this question, sharing what you feel you would like for dinner in a matter of seconds, and not thinking for fifteen minutes about what you think I want.

2. "A mirror."

3. If you say, "It's me," or describe some role you play, you will be told to come back when you know who you are. When you do not separate yourself from the divine, you might say, "It's you," or "Your child is here." Then you are invited in. The best answer I ever heard was from an obviously loved high school student: "Tell God his replacement is here."

Decades ago, psychiatrist Bruno Klopfer used the personality profiles from twenty-four cancer patients to predict who would have either a slow or a rapidly growing cancer. With five patients, he either was wrong or couldn't predict, but he was right twenty times. Psychiatrist Caroline Thomas at Johns Hopkins had medical students fill out a personality profile and draw a picture of themselves. She looked them up many years later, and from their personality profile and drawing, she was able to correlate and predict what diseases they would get and in which parts of their body. She hadn't thought cancer would have any psychological factors, and was truly surprised by her results.

One of Thomas's factors for predicting cancer was "a low closeness to parent profile." Similarly, a study of Harvard students revealed that of those who claimed that their parents did not love them, over 90 percent suffered a major illness by midlife, while those who felt loved by their parents had only one-fourth the illness rate of those who felt unloved. Today I see this in the cancer support groups and senior groups I run. The vast majority of participants feel loved, or they wouldn't be alive and fighting for their lives.

I also see people who accept their mortality and spend their remaining days doing what makes them happy. There was a man in London who was told he had two months to live. He went home and spent his last penny enjoying the time he had left and then felt fine and now wants to sue his doctor for making a mistake. Death is not a failure, though doctors rarely, if ever, use the words "dead" or "death." They talk about failing, passing, losing, moving on, and use expressions that keep them from discussing death. It is not an accident that most people in the hospital die at night, when doctors and loved ones are not present to interfere and create feelings of guilt. One doctor wrote an article, "Not on My Shift," about himself and two other young doctors who made a competition out of avoiding death by keeping a dying man from dying on their eight-hour shift. The one who wrote the article finally realized how sick their actions were.

I have also learned that death is not the worst outcome. One source of that belief is the words I quoted of author William Saroyan, who describes a young man dying and becoming, "dreamless, unalive, perfect." That is an accurate description of death. When you leave your body, you do not take your afflictions with you.

I have helped many people complete their lives by sharing their love and feelings and being able to die surrounded by their loved ones, and knowing they have not failed because their love is permanent and immortal. The deaths of my parents and my wife's parents have been shared with loved ones, peaceful and free of conflict. When they were tired of their bodies, they let us know. As my father-in-law said, and the words on his headstone explain, "He just fell up." When love is involved and conflict is resolved, you can turn off the "live" switch and do as he did. He refused his dinner and vitamins that night, let his loved ones know why, and died that evening. So I help people to live and die when they feel the time is right and their bodies are no longer a place they'd like to be.

Do I grieve? Yes, of course, but I have learned to live as they would want me to and not grieve excessively or uncontrollably so that my grief controls my life. Everyone in heaven carries a candle, and the only thing that can put it out I learned from my Dad after he died. In a dream, I was visiting him in heaven and saw his candle was out. When I offered to light it, he said, "They do but your tears keep putting it out." The lesson he taught me has been with me always. I recently expanded this into an illustrated children's book called *Buddy's Candle*.

Thankfully, I see some of the things I have just discussed becoming a standard part of medical care. Good progress, but it should have been done decades ago. We are just beginning to humanize medical care, as I would like to see it. I am also thrilled to see us moving ahead with therapy and technology. I envision the day that science will show us how to stop waging a war against cancer, thus empowering the disease with the focus upon war and conflict, and show us how to heal our lives and bodies. Harsh words such as "kill," "blast," "poison," and "assault" will be dropped from our medical language, stopping the perpetrating of negative hypnotic effects. Just read a chemotherapy protocol and you will see that it doesn't tell you about the benefits, it tells you about what will go wrong. Dave, a Quaker friend of mine, went to his oncologist and was told, "I am going to kill your cancer." Dave replied, "I'm a Quaker, I don't kill anything." He walked out of the office and drew a picture for me showing his white blood cells carrying the cancer cells away. He lived for over twelve years doing natural remedies.

I am sure the future of therapy will lie in communication with the patient, and between the patient and the cancer cell, and medications that will work in a natural way, on a genetic level, telling the cancer cell to die, stop reproducing, or revert to normal while the body's healthy cells remain undisturbed. This is similar to how bacteria, viruses, and plants have spontaneous, intelligent genetic changes and reversions to survive antibiotics, vaccines, and environmental changes. These changes are not lucky accidents. They happen quickly in response to the threat.

My hope is that cancer treatment of the future will heal lives and cure diseases. Acceptance of one's mortality can be a great teacher about life. As Elida Evans wrote in her book, *Psychological Study of Cancer*, in 1926, cancer is a message for the patient to take another path in his life. Cancer is growth gone wrong.

This is why I ask people to draw their treatment, so I can see what their inner wisdom will reveal. Some people who do not want chemotherapy draw a beautiful picture because their intuition knows it is right for them. Others are getting chemotherapy, and wonder why they are having so many side effects until they see the picture looks like hell. There are drawings of the operating room where God, love, and an unmasked surgeon are embracing the patient, and others where there is no one there to observe or care for the patient. Radiation therapy can be seen as a gift radiating from God, or as a threatening monster; so can eating vegetables. When love is combined with faith, hope, and joy, incredible results follow. I could tell from the drawings children did of themselves in the OR whether they were loved or not. Those who felt loved drew the operating room in natural, vibrant colors. Those who felt they were being operated upon as punishment by unloving parents drew a black, desolate room.

Your reaction will vary based upon your relationship with and belief in your treatment and your doctor. One word of advice from a group member: whenever a doctor prescribes something, always say no. Why? Because when you say no, the doctor realizes you are not a typical submissive sufferer. You are a *respant*. "Respant" is a word I created to represent a responsible participant, whom the doctor must sit down with and talk to so that the correct treatment decisions are made.

What needs to be treated is not just the cancer, but also the patient's experience. As I have said, technology is wonderful, but treatment must be of the individual and not just of the disease alone. When you ask people what they are experiencing, they do not answer with their medical diagnosis. They answer with feeling words such as "failure," "roadblock," "burden," "draining," and "sucking," but also with feeling words such as "blessing," "wake-up call" and "new beginning." What they are talking about is their life experience, which needs to be healed, because when you heal a life you also increase the likelihood of curing a disease. Healing is self-induced and not just about the somatic aspects of a patient's life. When I operate upon a person's body, I do not have to give that person a list of things to do in order to heal. The body knows, so we can cover a wound with a bandage and the body does what it needs to do.

Yes, there are ways to impede or enhance healing related to your feelings and life experience, because your internal chemistry is altered by your feelings. Our body loves us, but do we love our bodies and ourselves? When a woman described to me the experience of her disease as a failure, I asked her how that fit her life. She said, "Oh, my body failed me." I said, "I am asking about how the word fits your life." She answered, "My parents committed suicide when I was a child. So I must have been a failure as a child." Then we began to heal her life and cure her disease.

Alexander Solzhenitsyn, himself a survivor of cancer, says it all very well in his book *Cancer Ward*. He writes about the men sitting in the ward, and one is reading a medical textbook. He reads about cases of actual healing, not recovery though treatment. We generally hear doctors use the term "spontaneous remission" rather than "healing" when a patient gets well who is not expected to. What can we learn from a spontaneous remission? Not much. But we can learn a great deal from a case of self-induced healing.

Solzhenitsyn symbolizes it all beautifully and accurately. It is as though self-induced healing flutters out of the great open book like a rainbow-colored butterfly and the men in the ward all hold up their cheeks for its healing touch as it flies past. Only the gloomy Poduyev croaks out, "I suppose for that you need to have a clear conscience."

Solzhenitsyn is telling us that healing relates to transformation, as symbolized by the butterfly. The caterpillar dissolves and the butterfly is born and must struggle to leave the cocoon and survive. The rainbow represents our emotions. Every color represents an attitude or emotion. I see this every day in my work with drawings. When they form a rainbow, they reveal that your life is in order and you have a clear conscience and are living your true authentic life, not a role. You have found self-love and your divinity, as well as your faith, hope, joy, and a clear conscience, in the here and now.

I see life as a labor pain of self-birth, and that includes cancer treatment. I have seen many poems describing that view, and one compares the nine months of pregnancy to twelve months of chemotherapy and radiation. The former experience is worthwhile because you give birth to your child, and the latter is worthwhile because you give birth to yourself. Think of yourself as a blank canvas upon which you create a work of art by working and reworking with your brush and palette of colors. Survivors don't just fill their prescriptions; they think about their choices and make their own decisions.

There are many components of the survivor personality, including spiritual faith, and faith in your doctor, in your treatment, and in yourself. Hope is also an important component. I am reminded again of the lines by Emily Dickinson, "Hope is the thing with feathers, that perches in the soul, and sings the tune without the words, and never stops at all." She also wrote, "Surgeons must be very careful, when they take the knife! Underneath their fine incision, stirs the culprit—*Life!*"

Hope is always real and makes living more joyful. Please understand, there is no false hope. It is not about statistics, it is about possibilities and uncertainties. I know people who have left their troubles to God and had their cancer disappear. I don't recommend it as the only therapy because it isn't easy to do, but I have seen it happen more than once. God can also send a surgeon to help you. However, it shows how powerful faith and hope are; and when they are combined with peace of mind, some remarkable things can happen. When an authority figure tells you what is going to happen, it is hypnotic and can induce the results described. I knew a man who had lung cancer. When he developed cataracts, his health plan refused to pay for the surgery, claiming he would be dead soon and there was no point in wasting money on cataract surgery. The loss of his vision took the joy out of his life, which included playing with his grandchildren, reading the sports page of his newspaper, and betting on horse races. When the doctor denied his request for cataract surgery, he went home, climbed into bed, and died in a week.

That is why doctors need to be trained in communication and consider their patients' requests. I have seen the power of my words with children particularly. I would rub their arm with alcohol and tell them they would not feel the needle because of what I was rubbing on their arm. I deceived people into health at times. One-third of the children had local anesthesia induced by my words and were thrilled by the result. The others would tell me it didn't work but they still had less pain. I've even had children fall asleep being wheeled into the operating room and realized it was because I told them they would go to sleep in the OR. I even had to explain to some of them that I couldn't reach their appendix if they turned over and slept on their stomach.

We cannot survive without hope and meaning. Endless studies show that optimists have better health and longer lives than pessimists, even if they are less accurate about the reality of life. Many studies have come out showing that our feelings have physical consequences. Loneliness affects the genes, which control immune function. Cancer patients who laugh live longer. Treating depression with counseling and group meetings helps survival. How we feel is creating our chemistry.

People who volunteer also have better health, especially when they have a disease and are helping others with the same affliction.

In one study of cancer patients, the best survival rates were among those with a fighting spirit. Next came the deniers whose hope, in a sense, came from denying what could happen. The worst survival rates were in the hopeless, helpless group. One man was told he was HIV-positive and went home and developed all the symptoms. He'd had friends who had died of AIDS, so he knew the routine. Some months later, his doctor discovered there was a mistake in the report and he was HIV negative. When he heard about the mistake, he recovered his health in two short weeks.

I think what helped prepare me most for this work were the children I cared for. I'm reminded of a child whose dog was about to be euthanized, who said, "They have shorter lives because they don't need all the time it takes us to learn about love and forgiveness." Children and animals are my teachers because they teach us about living in the moment, having a sense of humor, not worrying about next week, asking for help, and sharing feelings. All of which are survival behavior qualities. It is painful to see a child die, and it has led me on a spiritual journey to try to understand and cope with this experience. I believe we are here on earth to become complete, and anything that helps us to do that is a blessing. The problem is that some blessings do not feel very good when they happen. What you may define as a curse can become a blessing if you let it become your teacher and show you that not all of the side effects of cancer are bad. I mentioned earlier how Lois Becker, a woman who wrote to me about her breast cancer, said, "Cancer made me take a look at myself and I like who I met."

So remember, the issue is: are you willing to be born again and again? As Martin Buber shared in his writings, if a woman goes into labor prematurely doctors treat her to stop her labor, but if she is in the ninth month they help her to deliver the child. Why not think of it this way: when you have a problem but are not ready or capable of change and being reborn, God steps in and answers your prayers. Not so, however, when it is time for you to be born again. Then it is time for you to change and God does not step in to solve the problem. It is now up to you. So again, this is not about God punishing you, instead it is about God giving you the opportunity to change through your efforts and labor pains and give birth to yourself.

I have studied many religions and found that some cause people to feel guilty when they develop an illness. However, for Jewish physician and philosopher Maimonides, disease was a loss of health, and we should all help the person to find their health again. A Muslim, after learning he had a serious illness, said, "All praise be to Allah." Why? Because he could see there would be a blessing associated with it. I know Christians who feel God gives them a disease to bring them closer to Him.

I am talking about self-love and the divinity within each of us. For me it is not about theology but about being a living example of faith, hope, joy, and love. This work has given me the gift of knowing so many inspiring people who have shown me what we are capable of surviving, and I do not mean that in the sense of being cured, but of living with the experience no matter how difficult it may seem. Faith, hope, joy, and love are what sustain us and can be our weapons as we kill with kindness and torment with tenderness. What we are here to do is live and learn, and the people who inspire me are my teachers and role models. William Saroyan, in *The Human Comedy*, wrote, "The best part of a good man stays . . . for love is immortal and makes all things immortal while hate dies every minute."

I am prepared for my own death and do not fear it or anything else. As one of our children e-mailed me when he was not having a good day, "Life sucks and most people suck and if you wake up one day and the world is beautiful and everyone loves one another, you're dead." So as I have said, for me death is not the worst outcome. I am not afraid that my life will end. I am more afraid it will never begin, and I try to live my life as if it were the last day of the lives of everyone I love. I hope you all can feel the same way and break out of the cocoon created by the words and actions of others and be transformed. Give your love to the world in the way you want to give it so you do not lose your life in order to please others.

At one point, I had three careers. All day I was the surgeon. Then, when I was done with surgery, I counseled people in the office every evening, and at home, I answered phone calls and letters every night. I realized I needed to focus and consolidate my life. I still meet people who were sustained by the fact that I wrote them a personal letter when they needed help. Today it is easier in some ways because of e-mails, but it also opens me to people from all over the world. So I am a busy man, but the gift is always in helping others. I never mind when people disturb me at home because I know they are survivors who have sought and found me. I have learned not to chase after and try to save them. When I help people find love, hope, joy, and faith, they benefit and so do I. I may get tired, but I am burning up and not out.

From my experience, I have learned to love myself and others, knowing that I am mortal and here for a limited amount of time. I also accept that I need to be coached by family, patients, and coworkers to become even more loving. I am ready to confess my weaknesses and defects while at the same time being grateful for life and the opportunity it provides.

I conclude with the words of Thornton Wilder in his book *The Bridge of San Luis Rey*: "And we ourselves shall be loved for a while and forgotten but the love will have been enough. All those impulses of love return to the love that made them. Even memory is not necessary for love. There is a land of the living and a land of the dying and the bridge is love, the only survival, the only meaning." So every day in my meditation and prayers, they are still with me and I do not let my tears put out their celestial candles because I know they want me to experience faith, hope, and joy.

Index